INDIAN DOCTOR BOOK

This is an example
of how early pioneers handled
their medical problems and
are in no way to be
construed for use as a
substitute to modern
medical techniques.

Distributed by Aerial Photography Services, Inc.
2511 South Tryon Street
Charlotte, North Carolina 28203
(704) 333-5143
ISBN 1-880970-76-7

INDIAN DOCTOR BOOK

Dedicated to
my Grandmother
Minnie Susan Decker
who used this book
second to the Bible
in the raising
of her
twelve children

Compiled and published by
Nancy Locke Doane

TABLE OF CONTENTS

POISONS.

1. Q. What is a poison?

A. A poison is any substance capable of altering or destroying some or all of the functions necessary to life.

2. Q. What are the principal mineral poisons?

A. Arsenic; antimony; copper; lead; and mercury.

3. Q. What are the symptoms of poisoning by arsenic?

A. An austere taste, constriction of the pharynx and esophagus, hiccup, nausea, and vomiting of brown or bloody matter; great anxiety; heat and severe pain at the pit of the stomach; black and foetid stools; small, frequent, and irregular pulse; palpitation, and difficult breathing; great thirst; burning heat; delirium, convulsions, and death.

4. Q. How is a case of poisoning by arsenic to be treated?

A. Vomiting is to be immediately excited by an emetic, of zinc, or ipecacuanha, aided by the liberal use of diluents. If vomiting is not speedily induced by these means, the stomach should be washed out by Jukes's syringe. After the stomach has been thus cleared of the poison, the next indication is to counteract the secondary symptoms. This is to be accomplished by venesection, fomentations, emollient glysters, as circumstances may require.

5. Q. Is there any known *antidote* to the poison of arsenic?

A. Sulphuret of potash, alkaline salts, charcoal, sulphur, & c., have all been recommended, but are of doubtful efficacy. Carbonate of magnesia is perhaps entitled to the most credit as an antidote.

6. Q. What are the tests of arsenic?

A. The following are the most important: viz.

1. The ammoniaco-nitrate of silver dropped into a solution of arsenic, produces a copious yellow precipitate, which in the course of a few hours turns to a dark brown.

2. The ammoniaco-sulphate of copper produces a copious green precipitate, well-known under the name of Scheele's green.

3. If a stream of sulphuretted hydrogen be passed through a solution of arsenic, it causes a yellow precipitate.

4. If arsenic be thrown upon hot coals, it burns with a garlic smell.

5. If arsenic be surrounded with a circle of charcoal, between two copper plates, and subjected to heat for a few minutes

on separating the plates a silver-like stain will be left upon the plates.

6. Another test is the reduction of the metal, but calcining the dried suspected matter in a glass tube, with equal parts of charcoal and potash, when, if arsenic be present, even in very minute quantity, it will be sublimed, in the form of a shining metallic coating.

7. Take a little recent wheat starch, add to it a sufficient quantity of *iodine* to give it a blue colour, mix a little of this blue matter with water so as to have a blue-colored liquid. If into this liquid a few drops of an aqueous solution of arsenious acid be put, the blue colour is immediately changed to a reddish brown, and is gradually dissipated entirely. If a few drops of sulphuric acid be now added, the blue colour is again restored.

8. Take a few drops of the solution of *chromate of potash* to the filtered solution, or to a grain of white arsenic in substance, and in half an hour a bright grass-green color will be produced.

7. Q. What are the appearances on dissection of a person who has been poisoned by arsenic?

A. The stomach is the principal seat of morbid appearances. The villous coat of that organ is most generally found in a state of high inflammation, frequently with erosions upon its surface. The intestines are also inflamed, but in a less degree. The lungs are also usually affected—they are livid, or have livid spots on their surface. The other viscera are generally in a healthy condition.

8. Q. What are the effects of a tart emetic, when taken in a large dose?

A. Severe pain in the stomach; excessive vomiting; profuse liquid stools; face pale; great prostration of strength; pulse small and feeble; cramps in the extremities.

9. Q. What are the appearances on dissection?

A. Inflammation of stomach and intestines. The lungs are also frequently inflamed.

10. Q. How is poisoning by tartar emetic to be treated?

A. Vomiting, if not already present, to be excited by tickling the throat with the finger or a feather, and dilating with large draughts of mild fluids. The inflammatory symptoms afterwards to be subdued by the usual antiphlogistic means.

11. Q. What are the best *antidotes* to tartar emetic?

A. Decoction of bark is the best. If this cannot be obtained, strong tea, or a decoction of nut galls, or any other astringent herb will answer.

12. Q. What are the tests of tartar emetic?

A. 1. Sulphuretted hydrogen and the hydro-sulphurets,

when used in small quantities, throw down an orange-yellow precipitate; when used in larger quantities, a deep brown-red.

2. Sulphuric acid produces a white precipitate.

3. Lime water, water of barytes, and alkalia give a thick white precipitate.

4. Infusion of galls causes a copious white precipitate, and is the most delicate test of all.

5. When heated red hot with the black flux, all the preparations of antimony are reduced to the metallic state.

13. Q. What is the preparation of copper which is most usually poisonous?

A. Verdegris, or the sub-acetate of copper.

14. Q. What are the symptoms of poisoning by copper?

A. An acrid, styptic, coppery taste in the mouth; parched and dry tongue; a sense of strangulation in the throat, coppery eructation, constant spitting, nausea, copious vomitings, or vain efforts to vomit, shooting pains in the stomach, which are often very severe; horrible gripings; frequent alvine evacuations, sometimes bloody and blackish, with tenesmus and debility; the abdomen inflated and painful; the pulse small, irregular, tight, and frequent; syncope, heat of skin, ardent thirst, difficulty of breathing, anxiety about the praecordia, cold sweats, scanty urine, violent headache vertigo, faintness, weakness in the limbs, cramps of the legs, and convulsions.

15. Q. What are the appearances on dissection?

A. The stomach and intestinal canal are found inflamed and sometimes gangrenous.

16. Q. How is poisoning by copper to be treated?

A. For the purpose of expelling the poison, vomiting is to be excited by copious draughts of milk and water. After this inflammatory symptoms are to be subdued by the usual means, and nervous symptoms by opium and antispasmodics.

17. Q. What is the antidote to copper?

A. Whites of eggs mixed up with water, which must be taken freely.

18. Q. What are the tests of verdegris?

A. 1. Mix the verdegris with charcoal, and heat it to redness in a crucible, and metallic copper will be formed.

2. Sulphuretted hydrogen precipitates a black sulphuret of copper.

3. Ammonia gives a blue precipitate, but if added in excess the precipitate re-dissolves, and the liquor is of a beautiful blue color.

4. A clean plate of iron immersed in the solution, becomes covered in a few hours with a portion of the copper, and the blue color of the solution grows first green, and then turns to red.

19. Q. What are the symptoms of poisoning by lead?

A. When taken in large quantities, a sweetish astringent, constriction of the throat, pain in the region of the stomach, obstinate and often bloody vomitings, hiccup, convulsions, and death.—When taken in small quantities and long continued doses, it causes colica pictorum and paralysis.

20. Q. What are the *antidotes* to lead?

A. Sulphate of soda and sulphate of magnesia.

21. Q. What is the treatment proper for cases of poisoning by lead?

A. A weak solution of Glauber's or Epsom salts to be drank very freely for the purpose of vomiting and purging, as well as to neutralize the poison.—Inflammatory symptoms to be afterwards subdued in the usual manner.

22. Q. What are the chemical tests of lead?

A. 1. All the preparations of lead are easily reduced to the metallic state by calcination with charcoal.

2. The *acetate of lead*, dissolved in water, is precipitated white by sulphuric acid.

3. By chromate of potash and chromic acid, it is precipitated of a canary-yellow color.

4. By sulphuretted hydrogen and the hydro-sulphurets, a black precipitate.

5. By sulphate of soda, a white precipitate.

6. Gallic acid gives a yellowish-white precipitate.

23. Q. What preparation of mercury is generally used as a poison?

A. The muriate of mercury, or corrosive sublimate.

24. Q. What are the symptoms of poisoning by corrosive sublimate?

A. An acrid, astringent, metallic taste in the mouth; stricture and burning in the throat; anxiety and rending pains in the stomach and intestines; nausea and vomiting, which is sometimes bloody; diarrhea, sometimes dysentery; pulse small, hard, and frequent; fainting; great prostration of strength; difficulty of breathing; cold sweats; cramps in the limbs; insensibility; convulsions, and death.

25. Q. What are the appearances on dissection?

A. Inflammation of the stomach and intestines, sometimes

ending in gangrene.

26. Q. What is the antidote to corrosive sublimate?

A. Albumen or the whites of eggs.—Lately wheat flour has been recommended.

27. Q. What is the treatment in cases of poisoning by corrosive sublimate?

A. The whites of eggs to be mixed with water, and one given every two or three minutes to promote vomiting as well as to decompose the poison. Milk, sugar and water, or water to be taken liberally at the same time. Symptoms of inflammation to be overcome by venesection, &c.

28. Q. What are the chemical tests of corrosive sublimate?

A. 1. By mixing corrosive sublimate with charcoal and water, and subjecting it to heat in a close vessel, metallic mercury is obtained.

2. By exposing it to heat without any admixture in a glass tube, it will be sublimed, and found lining the top of the tube in the form of a white shining crust.

3. By ammonia, a white precipitate is produced.

4. Carbonate of potash causes a precipitate like brick dust.

5. Caustic potash produces a yellow precipitate.

6. Lime water produces an orange-colored precipitate.

7. Nitrate of silver occasions a white curdy precipitate.

29. Q. What are the symptoms of poisoning by opium?

A. Stupor, numbness, heaviness in the head, pupil of the eye dilated, sometimes furious delirium, pain, convulsions of different parts of the body, or palsy of the limbs. The pulse is variable, but at first generally strong and full: the breathing is quick, and there is great anxiety, coma, death.

30. Q. What is the treatment in cases of poisoning by opium?

A. The stomach is first to be effectually evacuated, by emetica of tart; emetic or sulphate of zinc; large injections to clear the bowels, and assist in getting rid of the poison. When as much of the poison as possible has thus been expelled, the patient may drink, alternately, a tea-cup full of strong hot infusion of coffee and vinegar diluted with water. If the drowsiness and insensibility bordering on apoplexy be not remedied by these means, blood may be taken from the jugular vein, blisters may be applied to the neck and legs, and the attention roused by every means possible. If the heat declines, warmth and frictions must be perseveringly used. Vegetable acids are on no account to be given before the poison is expelled.

RECEIPTS.

No. 1.—FOR FEVER AND AGUE.

Take one pound of the bark of yellow birch, half pound sweet flag, half pound of tag alder bark, two ounces thorough wort, two ounces tanzy, dry, put to these four quarts of water, and boil slow, stir and boil the liquor down one half, then let it cool and add two quarts of sweet wine and bottle for use; dose one table-spoonful every two hours till the shake comes on, then no more that day, pursue this daily and you will be satisfied of its efficacy.

No. 2.—FOR GRAVEL.

Take horsemint, queen of the meadow, and clivers, equal parts, and boil in water down one half, and bottle for use; take one gill morning and evening, this effects a cure in about two months in the most obstinate cases.

No. 3.—FOR INTERNAL ULCERS.

Take one pound of blue flag, one of spignut, two ounces blood root, two ounces of coltsfoot, two ounces of Solomon's seal, two ounces of burdock seed, and one handful of peach kernels, boil these in four quarts of water three hours, then strain and add one pound loaf sugar, and one pint holland gin, take one tablespoonful three times each day, before eating; this is infallible.

No. 4.—FOR DROPSY.

Take four parts dwarf elder, three parts queen of the meadow, three parts of Jacob's ladder, three parts water or green briar, three parts of horseradish, two parts large or podded milkweed, boil them in sufficient water to cover them, then press out the li-quor, and add to every quart half pint of gin, it is then fit for use; take a wine glass full every four hours through the day. And the result will astonish you.

No. 5.—FOR CORNS.

Make a plaster of equal parts Canada balsam, and yolk of eggs, apply three times, it seldom fails curing the first application.

No. 6.—FOR DISPEPSIA.

Take two parts man root pulverized, two parts gum myrrh, two parts anis-seed, one part saffron, one part black alder bark, two parts orange peel, one part spignut, one part gentian, one part golden seal, and one part spearmint, all pulverized, put them all in a stone jug by the fire about blood warm six days, covered with brandy, or two quarts of brandy to one pound of the compound, then strain and add one pound of loaf sugar to every two quarts of liquor; dose one teaspoonful three times each day, or sufficient to operate on the bowels once in twenty-four hours, reduce the dose as the occasion requires, this is good in all disorders of the stomach, or liver, and is my panacea. This is worth fifty dollars to any family; it has cured thousands.

No. 7.—FOR INFLAMMATION OF THE STOMACH.

Take one part spignut, and one part bittersweet, and one part carrots boiled, apply external, then take one fourth ounce of lobe lia, one half ounce indian turnip, one half ounce of Solomon's seal, and a handful of marsh mallows, put them in one quart of pure spirits, twenty-four hours, and take as the stomach will bear. This is an excellent prescription and seldom fails.

No. 8.—FOR DIARRHEA OR FLUX.

First, take cordial, two scruples rhubarb, two of cinnamon, one of saleratus, one gill of boiling water, sweetened with loaf sugar, and one tablespoonful of best brandy. Second, syrup one part bayberry bark, one part cherry tree bark, one part white poplar bark, half part pond lilly, half part blackberry root, boil them and sweeten with loaf sugar, and a very little brandy. Third, injections, one pint mucilage of elm, one pint mucilage marsh mallows, one gill molasses, one pint sweet milk, half teaspoonful saleratus, and one fourth ounce of lady slipper. Fourth, wash the whole surface with saleratus and water, night and morning. Fifth, rubefacient to the bowels, one tablespoonful of spirits turpentine, and four of water, and four of brandy applied warm once in four hours, and a warm flannel bandage applied round the body. Directions, give one tablespoonful of the syrup every hour, and a teaspoonful of the cordial at the same time, until the evacuations are healthy, then continue the syrup alone, give an injection once in four hours, after applying the rubefacient to the bowels; for drink use mucilage of elm, or marsh mallows, and virginia snake root, or ginger. This is infallible.

No. 9.—FOR PILES.

If the piles are outward, make an ointment of fireweed, sage, parsley, mayweed, burdock, narrow dock, sweet elder and butter, simmered together, anoint the parts with this two or three times each day, and drink constantly a tea made by steeping the roots of burdock and narrow dock, as much as is convenient, but if they are inward or blind piles, apply the balsam of tamerack on cotton to the parts, and drink essence of fur every night. Infallible.

No. 10.—FOR OBSTRUCTED MENSTRUATION.

Take three parts of female flowers, commonly found by the side of ponds, leaf deep green, shapen like the cowslip, flowers of a bright yellow, this certainly is one of the first herbs in the world for females; two parts of unkum, found in swamps, known by the name of blood gut, and one part of Indian pink, boil them in fair water till the strength is all out, then strain and add to this as much port wine, or good madeira, as will keep it from souring, and take a wine glass full three times each day, if the bowels are costive, use a little syrup of elecampane, and I warrant you a speedy cure.

No. 11.—FOR ASTHMA

Take one ounce of lobelia seed, one ounce skunk cabbage root, one ounce of garlic, half a pound of seneca snake root, half a pound of spignut, half a pound of parsleyroot, one pound of liquorice root, and the liver of a sheep or calf, or wolf, boil them all in one gallon of sweet wine, and three gallons of rain water, till you reduce it one half, then bottle for use; dose half a tablespoonful, three times each day one hour before eating. This has cured hundreds.

No. 12.—FOR PLEURISY

Take one fourth of an ounce of lady slipper, one fourth of an ounce of red pepper, one fourth of an ounce of coriander seed, one and one fourth ounces of ginger, pulverize them all together; dose one teaspoonful every fifteen minutes till the pain subsides, this will generally be in one hour, take pleurisy root pulverised fine and steeped strong any quantity and take as the stomach will bear, till a sweat is brought on all over the body, then wear a flannel band around the abdomen a few days, and the cure is complete without weakening and debilitating the system by bleeding. This is infallible.

No. 13.—FOR MEASLES, CANKER RASH OR CHICKEN POX.

Take equal parts of queen of the meadow, white snake root, coltsfoot snake root, marigold and saffron, steep them together and drink plentifully through the progress of the disease; a vomit of equal parts of thoroughwort and lobelia, is necessary once in about three days, keep the body from exposures of cold or wet, and let the food be light and easy of digestion.

No. 14.—FOR THE SMALL POX

Take half a pound of saffron, half a pound of spignut root, one pound sassaparilla, one fourth of a pound of the seeds of young cedar, or one ounce of the oil of cedar, one fourth pound of sage and make into one mass, then steep strong as much as you think you can consume in one day in decoction, it is best made every day fresh as liquor of any kind is injurious and it will not keep longer in warm weather without spirits. This may be taken in any quantity and at any stage of the disease, and has never been known to fail when the patient is kept clean and warm. If the patient should by accident or imprudence take cold it is necessary to take 10 or 15 large onions, roast them, press the juice and let the patient drink the whole at once and apply the pressed pomice to the feet and he will soon be in profuse sweat. This is infallible.

No. 15.—FOR COSTIVENESS

Take equal parts of balmony, elecampane, spignut, gentian, ginseng, indian turnip, and tomatoes, boil them all in a quantity of fair water, boil it down to the consistency of new milk, then add one fourth quantity of good wine, and bottle for use; dose tablespoonful three times each day before eating. This is one of the best preparations in this Materia Medica.

No. 16.—FOR CHOLERA MORBUS.

Take equal parts of indian turnip, cayenne pepper, prickley ash berries, half part of spearmint, half part of horsemint, half part of bayberry bark, half part of sage, boil it in four quarts of water down one half, let it be well sweetened with loaf sugar, and a little brandy; dose half teaspoonful every half hour, till relief is obtained. The patient also ought to have an injection of slippery elm, with one fourth teacupful of the above in it. When this is strictly attended to, it never fails to relieve.

No. 17.—FOR CONSUMPTION.

This disease is one of the worst of diseases that attend the human frame, and is the most obstinate to subdue, and for this reason there are many old women and quacks prescribing specifics for it, but when tested prove inefficient for the malady, the patient generally sinks under the most skillful treatment when deeply seated. I believe the only remedy is death, but as we are all anxious to try every means when death stares us in the face, I give you the following for trial, it has cured many diseases of the breast and lungs, but I believe it never cured the consumption when seated. Take first one part elecampane, one part spignut, one part sage, one part hoarhound, one part yellow parilla, one part golden seal, one part Solomon's seal, half part of gum myrrh, half part gum guiacum, half part tamerack gum, all boiled in rain water, then put one gill of wine to every pint, bottle up, and take one wine glass full three times each day, also take one quart of St. Croix rum, and one pint honey, allum the size of an egg, boil and skim as long as there is any froth, then bottle for use; dose one tablespoonful three times each day, with the above syrup.

No. 18.—FOR INFLUENZA.

Take one ounce of cinnamon, half ounce of cloves, half ounce of hemlock bark, half ounce of gum arabic, mix all together in one quart of boiling water, take half teacupful, three or four times an hour, till you are in a profuse sweat, then take less as the occasion requires. Make a mucilage of elm, or blue flag, and drink plentifully, also sweat the throat with sage and hops, bath the feet in saleratus, and vinegar, and keep warm. This is a good receipt and seldom fails.

No. 19.—FOR COUGHS.

Take one ounce of meadow cabbage, one ounce of lobelia, half ounce of indian turnip, one fourth ounce of blood root, handful of hoarhound, one fourth ounce of elecampane, and the weight of the whole of purified honey, pulverize the ingredients and mix them up, and let the patient take what the stomach will bear, till well.

No. 20.—FOR PALSY.

First let the patient thoroughly cleanse the blood with burdock root, then take one ounce of umbil, called lady slipper, half pound of angle worms, half pint of spirits turpentine, fourth of a pound of lobelia seed, one ounce oil origanum, one ounce oil of spruce, one ounce oil of cinnamon, four green frogs alive, put these all in a stone vessel, under a heap of rotten manure, well stopped up for ten days, then take it out and strain it, and rub the afflicted; parts with it, and wrap the parts in flannel as warm as can be borne, let the patient drink plenty of sage, pennyroyal, or horsemint tea, for a constant drink, and I warrant them a speedy cure.

No. 21.—FOR GOUT.

Take the buds of the balm of Gilead, and put them in alcohol, and apply to the affected parts, (inwardly,) take queen of the meadow roots one ounce, hemp one ounce, of spignut one ounce, steep them, and mix with one bottle of sarsaparilla syrup, take sufficient to keep the bowels laxative. This is certain.

No. 22.—FOR RHEUMATISM.

Take one ounce of cayenne pepper, four ounces of ginger, two ounces of cinnamon, two ounces of cloves, one ounce of gum guiacum, one ounce of gum myrrh, one gallon fourth proof spirits, let them stand by the fire ten days before bottling, then place them in corked vessels and take one wine glass full three times each day, before eating. Rubefacient for the surface, boil one pound of red pepper, in one gallon of vinegar and wash every night just going to bed, also wear flannel next to the skin continually.

No. 23.—FOR QUINSY.

First take a flannel cloth and wet it in strong boiling vinegar and apply it around the neck, repeat this as often as it gets dry, then take one pint of brewers yeast and let the patient take one tablespoonful every few minutes and gargle the mouth with the same, and swallow some; do this till the whole is gone and with it your quinsy will be gone.

No. 24.—FOR WHOOPING COUGH.

Take equal parts of elecampane, skunks cabbage, hoarhound, and spignut, and boil till you extract the strength, then strain and boil down again to the consistence of tar, then add twice its weight of pure honey, and put it in a warm oven till well baked, let the patient take half teaspoonful often through the day. This is sure.

No. 25.—FOR CROUP.

This is very fatal among children. The best remedy for it is, equal parts blood root, lobelia, garlic, skunks cabbage, elecampane, sage, and thorough wort, or seneca snake root, or if the whole cannot be had, lobelia tincture, will do alone, or lobelia, and mullen roots, in decoction, give as much as possible, as the stomach will immediately eject any of these articles in this disease.

No. 26.—FOR RICKETS.

Drink a strong tea of sage, and sweet fern, and sleep on a bed made of the same until well, wash often in saleratus and strong cider or vinegar.

No. 27.—FOR LIVER COMPLAINT.

Take equal parts of tomatoes, balmony, yellow poplar, spignut, saffron, cinnamon, nutmegs and queen of the meadow, make an extract of these and then pill with unicorn, take from three to five daily. Infallible.

No. 28.—FOR JAUNDICE.

Take equal parts of white snake root, burdock, narrow dock, dandelion and cowslip blows, steep them together and drink as much as you can till well. This is a sure cure.

No. 29.—FOR DIFFICULTY OF URINE.

Take clivers, queen of the meadow, gravel wort, water brier, and brook lime, steep them in boiling water, let them steep till all the strength is out, then let it cool and drink this for a constant drink. This will be certain it never fails.

No. 30.—FOR GLEET.

Take bloodroot, cocash, water brier, unkum, burdock, raspberry leaves, and white snake root, steep strong, and drink what the stomach will bear, for a wash take lobelia seed, gum myrrh, gum guiacum, and oil of cedar, put them in alcohol and use two or three times each day. Infallible.

No. 31.—FOR VENEREAL.

Take burdock, narrow dock, yarrow, knott grass, clivers, bloodroot, equal parts, half part of water brier, half part Jacob's ladder, half part wormwood, half part lobelia herb, boil all in rain water, so as to make one gallon about the consistency of new milk, then add as much sugar as will preserve it, and drink daily what the stomach will bear. If there is costiveness, take frequent doses of lime water, make a wash with the tincture of lobelia, and spirits of turpentine, use it often, take a new cloth every time, and never put the cloth in the wash, but pour the liquid on the cloth, and then after using throw it away, change the linen often, and this is a sure cure in the worst of cases.

No. 32.—FOR WHITES.

Make a syrup of unkum, bloodgut, knott grass, yarrow, house plantain, raspberry leaves, and rue, boil the whole in fair water, sufficient to extract the strength, then strain and add to each quart one pound loaf sugar, one pound pure honey, one pint port wine, and take two tablespoonsful three times each day before eating, steam the parts with a flannel soaked in liquor in which hazel leaves have been boiled, (that is water, understand,) apply this three or four times if the occasion requires.

No. 33.—FOR NERVOUS AFFECTIONS.

Take one ounce lobelia seed, one ounce cayenne, one ounce Solomon's seal, one ounce of blue violet roots, one ounce of spignut, two ounces of yellow poplar, handful beech drops, the same quantity of Indian pipe or fit root, put the whole in four quarts of pure Holland gin, by the fire, lightly corked seven days, then strain and add four pounds of molasses, or brown sugar, and pour two quarts of rain water, bottle for use. This is infallible.

No. 34.—FOR ULCERS ANY WHERE ON THE BODY.

Wash the complaining parts with lobelia tincture every day, and make an ointment of green frogs, shrub, maple, spignut root, gumfrey, white elder bark, and blue flag root, two ounces of each, to four green frogs, first steep the roots, barks and herbs in two pounds of hogs lard, then strain after boiling, and apply this daily to the ulcer; and the effect will astonish you.

No. 35.—FOR SORES.

Take male hogs lard one pound, spignut half pound, fourth of a pound of Solomon's seal, the extract of dandelion one ounce, the seed of lobelia one ounce, one ounce of spirits turpentine, four ounces rosin, two ounses beeswax; and make it into a salve, and apply till well.

No. 36.—FOR SCROFULA.

Cleanse the blood with burdock, and black alder bark, and tag alder bark, and sassafras bark and wash the surface with tincture of tony weed, and brewer's yeast, dry the parts well after using. This is simple and sovereign.

No. 37.—FOR CLEANSING THE BLOOD.

Take burdock roots brush them clean, and slice them up, and put them in cold water, and drink for common, or take yellow dock, and boil it in water, and drink half pint each day, or take a decoction of sassafras for a common drink, or black alder bark, or tag alder bark, or cucumber bark, or yellow poplar bark, in decoction, these are all very good and are best when used alternately.

No. 38.—FOR PAIN IN THE SIDE.

Make a plaister of the balsam of Canada, or tamerack, and wear on the side, and drink a tea made of bittersweet and celandine. Infallible.

No. 39.—FOR PROLAPSUS UTERI.

First let the patient be placed as near as possible in an horizontal position, and remain as much as is convenient in that position for eight to ten days, during which time there must be steeped in water, witch hazel leaves, and slippery elm, and flannel cloths wet this liquor, applied to the parts as often as they cool, they must be as warm as can be borne, the patient must take as much beth root, pulverized as will fill a teaspoon, three times each day in half teacuful of the same liquor, also a free drink of either, or all of the articles under the head of the receipt for cleansing the blood, the patient's food must be light soups, or mucilages, till the cure is effected, drastic purges must be avoided always.

No. 40.—FOR THE ITCH.

Take one pound of burdock root green, one pound of, yellow-dock root, and tops green, boil them in two quarts of water one hour, then strain, and add fourth of a pound of hogslard, two ounces of sulphur, four ounces of spirits of turpentine, then boil again to the consistency of tar, wash all over first, then rub it in well by the fire just before going to bed, repeat this three times, and then change your clothes and keep clean. This never fails.

No. 41.—FOR ST. ANTHONY'S FIRE.

Take equal parts of tory weed, lobelia herb, witch hazel, knott grass, and tag alder bark, green or dry, boil them strong, and wash the complaining parts, and let the patient drink at intervals a little syrup of sarsaparilla. This is an immediate cure.

No. 42.—FOR FEVER.

First take an emetic of lobelia, accompanied with stimulants so as to cause free perspiration, then relieve the bowels with some mild physic, bitterroot is as good as any, this is the small milk-weed, take one tablespoonful of the powdered root in a little water, and repeat as often as necessary till the evacuations are healthy. If the fever is not entirely broke, you must repeat the above, then make some bitters with yellow poplar, balmony, and black cherry bark, in wine, or gin; this is the best way to cure fevers, as it neither needs the lancet, nor calomel; and is perfectly safe.

No. 43.—FOR WHEEZING OR SHORTNESS OF BREATH.

Take one ounce of skunk cabbage root dry, one ounce of mullen root dry, and half pound of liquorice root, put them all in two quarts of Malaga wine or sweet wine, and exercise moderately.

No. 44.—FOR WIND IN THE STOMACH.

Take equal parts of unicorn root, Indian turnip and prickley ash berries, and pulverize them and take one teaspoonful in a little liquor, and it is a very sure cure, or take one ounce of each of the above and put in one quart of gin and take as occasion requires.

No. 45.—FOR LOSS OF APPETITE.

Make a syrup with equal parts, white and black cohosh, half a part golden seal, half a part of bitter root, half a part of columbia root, and put sufficient liquor in it to preserve it. This restores the appetite in debilitated cases.

No. 46.—FOR PAIN OR CHOLIC IN THE BOWELS.

Take cayenne pepper, cloves, unicorn, dogwood bark, and prickly ash berries, equal parts or a half part of the cayenne and put them all in spirits sufficient to cover them, they will be fit to use the second day after making, or boil the bottle that has them in with the liquor one hour, and they may be used; take one tablespoonful at a dose in a little water, repeat as often as necessary. This is also good for the pleurisy, there is no danger if you use a dose every ten minutes, if the pain is not reduced follow up till it is, then take physic.

No. 47.—FOR BLEEDING AT THE LUNGS.

Make a syrup with one ounce of red beth root, half an ounce of bayberry root in some water, in which witch hazel leaves have been boiled in, one pint, then add half a pint of good wine and sugar, or honey, and take one tablespoonful every ten minutes till it abates or ceases, then take half a pint of yeast and boil it with the same quantity of balsam of tamerack and take one tablespoon night and morning for ten days, sure cure.

No. 48.—FOR CANKER IN THE MOUTH.

Take golden seal, gold thread, elecompane roots, equal parts, then pulverize them and take one ounce of the mixture, and put to it one ounce of alum pulverized and the whites of four eggs, then put them into a mortar and mix them well, and take a little in the mouth and keep moving it round till it is all decomposed, then wash the mouth and repeat once an hour; it is also necessary to take an emetic to cleanse the stomach.

No. 49.—FOR WORMS.

Take one ounce of wormwood, one ounce of elecompane, half an ounce of lobelia, one ounce of tamarack, balsam, and one ounce of sage, put the whole in one pint of spirits of turpentine and half a pound of honey; these articles must stand in blood warm heat, for one or two days, then pressed out and they are fit for use; one teaspoonful every hour for four hours for a child of five years old, is a proper dose in sweet milk, and varied according to the age: it is best to give this in the morning and then directly after give a dose of Castor Oil and the worms must be carried away if there is any.

No. 50.—FOR POLYPUS IN THE NOSE.

Wash the external parts with the tincture of lobelia daily, and make a snuff with equal parts blood root, ginger, lobelia seed, and cloves, and this will kill the polypus, then pull it out, and syringe the parts with the tincture of lobelia, or mullen, until well.

No. 51.—FOR SHRUNK SINEWS OR STIFF JOINTS.

First put in a copper vessel, one layer of hogslard, and then one layer of wormwood, then again a layer of hogslard, then a layer of tanzey, then again the lard, then a layer of green melolet, then again the lard, then a layer of Bittersweet bark, then again the lard; then cover the whole tight with a lid, or a plate, let them simmer four hours, then strain, and apply first the dregs in two separate parts to the joints affected, and the one above till it becomes cold, then throw it away, and add to your ointment four green frogs, and half pint spirits turpentine, and again boil four hours and strain, then bind on the frogs as before directed, by this time your ointment will be sufficiently cool to use, the ointment must be applied to the affected joint, and the one above, for a month or more if necessary. This will perform a cure in almost any case, keep the bowels open during the treatment with laxitives.

No. 52.—FOR BLEEDING AT THE NOSE.

Take birthroot, and cranesbill, pulverized, and snuff this up the nostrils, and I warrant you a speedy cure. They must be gathered and dried, then pulverized and mixed, and kept constantly on hand where there are persons afflicted with this simple disease, which sometimes proves fatal.

No. 53.—FOR KINGS EVIL.

This disease may be cured with the plant by the same name, it grows in moist shady land, under almost all kinds of timber through the United States, it is something like plantain, but the leaves are smaller, spotted green and white, it is a beautiful plant, when it goes to seed there is one stalk which comes up in the middle of the plant, about nine inches high, it carries the seed in a small round bud at the top take the whole of it, root, leaves, and top, and pound it soft, apply to the tumor the poultice, when it is broke apply the salve made from the same with balsam of fir, and male hogs lard, wash the parts in a strong decoction of the same daily, and drink of the tea night and morning. And this will never fail.

No. 54.—FOR SPITTING BLOOD.

Make a decoction of cranesbill, birthroot, and gill-go-by-the-ground, equal parts, steep them strong, and drink as often as three or four times each day, this is cooling, abstersive, and vulnerary, and is the best compound for this complaint in the world.

No. 55.—FOR HYSTERICS.

Take a quantity of mountain tea, white root, and unkum root, equal parts, pound them, and make them into pills with Canada balsam, and yellow poplar, take two or three of these pills when the disorder is coming on; it seldom fails to arrest it in its progress.

No. 56.—FOR CANKER RASH.

Pulverize white birthroot, and give the patient small doses, four or five times each day, for the fever give sage, or pennyroyal tea, with some laxitive medicine. This is an excellent remedy.

No. 57.—TO STOP A FEVER SORE FROM COMING TO A HEAD, AND CARRY IT AWAY.

Sweat it with flannel cloths, dipped in hot brine, the cloths must be changed as often as they get cold for three hours, and then washed in alcohol, and bound in flannel, repeat this five or six times, and then take shrub-maple, and drink some of the decoction, and wash with the same, burdock roots shaked in cold water, are very good to purify the blood, and assist in curing this disease.

No. 58.—TO CURE A WEN.

Take one pound of lead, and boil it in one quart of water, then take the whites of eggs, and mix with it, and make into ointment, bind this on the wen with a cotton cloth. This will certainly cure the wen.

No. 59.—FOR LOCK JAW.

When a person is taken with the lock jaw, give from half a teaspoonful of the pulverized bud of lobelia, with the same quantity of Indian turnip, in a little warm water, repeat this every fifteen minutes, place the feet in a tub of warm water, and wash the head with the stimulating linament, then after the operation of the lobelia, place them in a warm bed, and place a hot stone to the feet wrapped in wet flannel, and the same to his side. This never fails, repeat if necessary.

No. 60.—TO STOP PUKING.

Give the patient as much poland starch, as he can conveniently take, or take a handful of grass, pound it fine, and put water to it, and let it be pressed; and give the patient as much as a gill once in half an hour, repeat till you have accomplished your object. The first is the best remedy in the world.

No. 61.—A SURE REMEDY FOR WOMENS SORE NIPPLES.

When the infant stops sucking, apply a plaister of Canada balsam, or balm of tamerack; this cures in less than a week, or apply the tincture of lobelia, as a wash to the breast, or wild cabbage leaves, over the fire, and put half a dozen on the breast at a time, steep it three or four times.

No. 62.—FOR CONVULSION FITS.

Take any quantity of Indian pipe, steep and drink as much as the stomach will bear three or four times a day, then make a syrup of the same, and sweeten with sugar, and take a wine glass full every morning. This is an Indian remedy, and well approved by all who have seen it used.

No. 63.—FOR STOPPAGE OF WATER.

Take a quantity of water brier, Jacob's ladder, queen of the meadow, parsley, and horse radish; put them in old cider, and drink a glass three or four times a day.

No. 64.—FOR APOPLEXY.

The tincture of nicotianne drawn with rectified French brandy, may be given to the patient, which instantly causes a great quantity of mucos to come out of the head, and afford a considerable relief, particularly if the remedy is repeated two or three times.

One can also give the extract of balm mint, from one scruple to one drachm; or the water of the same plant, from two to six ounces.

Likewise real queen Hungary water, from one to two drachms; or spirits of wine, from one to three drachms, do not less relieve the patient.

No. 65.—BALSAM TO CURE SORES.

Take some flowers and leaves of hypericum or St. John wort, of valerian, of sage, and of the two sorts of aristolochy round and long, about the same quantity of each; add to it a sufficient quantity of oil of turpentine or oil of roses, and boil the whole on a slow fire during one hour, afterwards, strain and press your balsam, and put it into a glass or earthen vessel and use the same when required.

No. 66.—BALSAM TO EASE PAINS.

You must take nettles and plantain leaves, and of the large daisy, of each three handfuls, with ten pounds of oil of acorn, and two quarts of the best white wine; put the whole together into a glass vessel, after having well pounded the herbs in a mortar, and having covered the vessel, put it to infuse on some hot ashes during twenty-four hours, and then cook it on a slow fire, until the wine is almost consumed; then strain and press well your balsam, and keep it as above to make use of in liniment for all kinds of pains.

No. 67.—BALSAM FOR ALL KINDS OF PAINS.

Take laurel leaves, wormwood sprouts, marigold flowers and leaves, of each two handfuls, cut them all very fine, sprouts of fine sage and of rosemary flowers and leaves, of each three handfuls, and eight handfuls of juniper berries; put the whole in glazed earthen pot, and after having poured over it a quantity of sweet oil so as the cover the whole about an inch, cause it to infuse amongst some very hot horse dung, during several days, then you will cook it over a very slow fire, and after it is done, you must add to it a small quantity of new yellow bees wax, a small glass of brandy, and one dozen of cloves; stir well the whole, and let it take a little boiling over the fire, and then strain it through a strong linen, pressing the ground well, and keep it for use in an earthen pot.

No. 68.—A CATAPLASM TO RESOLVE ALL SORES AND TUMORS.

Take one handful of grape vine branch ashes, which you will put to infuse into a pint of good white wine over hot ashes during fifteen or sixteen hours. In this colature, dilute a small handful of rye meal with the bran in, to make with it a kind of mush. Spread this cataplasm on a red cabbage leaf past over the fire, of the like size of the afflicted part, and apply over it a warm cloth in several folds.

No. 69.—FOR SWELLINGS AND INFLAMMATIONS.

Take one pint of good wine, some crumbs of white bread, or such as you can get, and a spoonful of oil of sage; make with the whole a mush, which you will apply hot two or three times a day. When it is to apply to a sore breast, the oil of roses is not necessary.

No. 70.—TO CAUSE SORE BREASTS TO OPEN.

Take two handfuls of sorrel, put it into an earthen pot, with a piece of fresh butter of the size of an egg, one or two spoonfuls of verjuice. Boil the whole together, until it is done, take it from the fire, and put into it some leaven of the size of two walnuts, when it is no more than lukewarm, take a little of it, and apply on the sick part, after having previously greased it with oil of roses, and change it three times a day. You must never break the sore when it is on the breast, but let it break itself.

No. 71.—TO APPEASE PAINS.

Take some soot, white of eggs, and a little oil of roses, beat the whole together, and make of it a cataplasm. Or else,

Take some good bran, flax-seed, beer, oil of camomile and melilot, with which you will make your cataplasm.

No. 72.—FOR ALL KINDS OF SWELLINGS.

Take half a pound of the meal of Windsor beans, two handfuls of well pounded wheat bran, two handfuls of ox dung, worm wood leaves, cammomile flowers and melilot, one handful and a half, oil of roses, and of aniseed of each two ounces, clear lye of ashes as much as will be necessary; the whole well pounded and put to boil altogether, and stir it until it thickens, you will then spread it on tow, and apply it warm to the afflicted part, and change it twice a day, until a cure takes place.

No. 73.—FOR PAINS AND SWELLINGS.

Take some Provinse roses, port wine, wheat bran and oil of roses, and make of it a cataplasm, and apply it as warm as you can bear it on the sick part.

No. 74.—FOR COMPLAINTS ABOUT THE EARS.

This complaint is a swelling that comes under the ears and that goes down to the neck; here are the remedies to cure it. Take a lily oignons and cut it, then cook it with half a glass of oil of violet, and the same quantity of wine, until the wine is consumed, afterwards throw into it half a handful of marsh mallows cut fine, the yellow of an egg and some rye flour, until the whole be capable of forming a cataplasm, to be applied warm on the disease; it must be changed three times, then the patient must be bled. Lilly oil with some black sheep's wool, is also proper for it. It is also necessary to purge the patient with glisters.

No. 75.—FOR SORE BREASTS.

Take one spoonful and a half of rye flour, which you will dilute with a gill of white wine, let it boil three or four bubblings, then take it off the fire, and put into it a large handful of ashes of the branches of grape vine, a little tallow, and a little of turpentine of Venice. Boil it again three or four bubblings, and stir it constantly until it be of a consistency to make cataplasms. This causes the sore to open, without being obliged to make use of the lancet. Hereafter, and in the article of plaster, will be found other remedies, to ripen and resolve a posthumed breast, and for other complaints of the same.

No. 76.—FOR CANCERS.

Take a large red onion, roast it well, take pocoon root finely powdered, mix this powder of the root with the onion, which must be well beaten, in the proportion of a teaspoonful to one onion: make of this a plaster just large enough to cover the sore. If really a cancer, this will produce great pain, yet the patient must not be alarmed, but repeat this every twelve hours, until the body of the cancer assumes a deep purple or black colour. Two plasters will generally effect this. The next preparation is this:

Take young poke root roasted, one handful, add one spoonful Jamestown seed powdered, about the same quantity of boars tusk root; (this root ought to be kept soaked in water;) beat these well together, then moisten this compound with the water from which the root is taken, and apply it night and morning. This is for the purpose of drawing out the cancer. Care must be taken not to force it out only as the plaster itself effects it, as much an operation would tend to break the small roots before they are entirely killed. If they are not entirely destroyed it may be known in eight or ten days as inflammation will take place; in such a case, the first preparation may again be used, and continue to be used once in ten days, until all the roots are destroyed, then the plaster will heal the sore.

Any careful person may perform the cure of cancers by a strict attention to the above directions.

No. 77.—ANOTHER FOR CANCERS.

Another evidence of the efficacious quality of pipsissiway in curing cancers. James Lewis, of this country, has called upon me, and wishes me to make known, that he was cured of a very large and painful cancer, by the use of pipsissiway tea, a strong decoction of the same which he applied to the sore, in the space of three weeks time; the cancer was on his cheek, the scar of which is still visible, and shows it to have increased to an alarming degree. He likewise affirms that it will cure other eruptions.

No. 78.—FOR WINDY CHOLIC.

Take acorn oil, from two drachms to one ounce, or else the acorn itself grated with its shell, likewise from one to four scruples, which will wonderfully relieve the patient from pains, by dissipating all winds that caused them. It is to be taken in a glass of white wine. Some nutmegs grated in broth, affords a great relief, or oil of aniseed from one to six drops.

No. 79.—FOR BILIOUS AND WINDY CHOLIC.

Take twelve or fifteen leeks, cut them into bits, put them in a kettle and cook them in a quart of vinegar, during three or four hours; when they are done, take them up with a skimmer, and apply them with your hand, on the skin where the pain lies, and towards the heart; dip afterwards, a napkin, which you will fold in four double, in the vinegar that has remained in the kettle, and put it over the said leeks; bind the whole with another dry napkin, and you will keep yourself laying on your back during two hours; after which you will take a glyster with honey.

No. 80.—FOR NEPHRITIC CHOLIC, PHLEGMS, SAND, STONE IN THE REINS, OR IN THE BLADDER, OR OTHER COMPLAINTS.

Take nephritic wood the weight of two ounces, which is sold by druggists, cut it in the finest and thinnest manner possible, and put it in a small glass bottle, pour over it some of the best brandy made of wine, until it covers the said nephritic wood, three good fingers breadth: leave it in infusion during three or four days until the brandy has entirely drawn the virtue of said wood; and whenever any person is attacked with the accidents common to that disease, as extraordinary swellings of the belly with pains, pains about the reins and ureters, or inclination to vomiting, take finger's breadth in a glass of that infusion, which will much relieve; but if the complaint be too tenacious apply over the region of the ureters some small bags filled with pellitory boiled in white wine; nevertheless, without the help of these said small bags, the virtue of this infusion will manifest itself, by the ejection that will take place with the urine, that will be thick and of a greyish cast, and sometimes mixed with sand, gravel or stone that caused the pain. This remedy may be repeated more than once in order to obtain more relief.

No. 81.—FOR CHOLERA-MORBUS.

Every year being extremely fatal to children, as such numbers of them have been swept away by the flux and cholera, or vomiting and purging; the following remedy for the cure of these diseases will be acceptable. Take oil of peneroyal, two drops to a tablespoonful of molasses, after being well stirred up, let one teaspoonful be administered every hour until it has the desired effect, which from experience, I can assure safely the public, will be found in every case of the above disorder to be a speedy and certain cure. For a grown person the dose may be doubled and given in the same manner.

No. 82.—ANOTHER.

Toast or brown in a vessel, as you would coffee, four tablespoonfuls of oatmeal, pour on it a pint of boiling water, add a little sugar to make it agreeable.

If the child is not too young, let it drink of it, grounds and all stirred up together. It is believed that this toasted oat meal tea is scarcely ever ejected from the stomach, on which it lies light, and to which it proves exceedingly grateful. For the information of the poorer class of citizens it is requisite to mention that oat meal can be procured at any of the druggists' shops.

No. 83.—FOR CRACKED HANDS.

In the first place wash your hands in warm water, then rub on common soap thoroughly, and scour your hands about two minutes with house ashes; then wash them again in warm water. This repeated a few times will effect a cure and keep the hands soft and pliable.

No. 84.—FOR DIARRHEA AND COMPLAINT OF THE BOWELS.

In case of a bilious diarrhea, one may make use with a happy success during a few days in the mornings, of a dose prepared with two ounces of the oil of sweet almonds, one ounce of lemon juice, and four ounces of plantain water.

Distilled water of acorn, impregnated with its fixed salt, and often given to the patient at the weight of two ounces, with one ounce of red poppy syrup; stop in a short time, not only the lax, but also (in women) the whites and excessive menstruous flux. One may also make use of the greatest part of the remedies proper to the following sickness.

No. 85.—FOR THE DYSENTERY.

Take of walnut oil extracted without fire, two ounces, the same quantity of rose water, beat them well together, and give to the patient in the morning fasting, two hours afterwards, he must take a bowlfull of boiled milk, with salt or sugar, and he will receive a quick relief from it.

No. 86.—FOR DROPSY.

Take about two large teacups full of Bohea tea, infuse it in a quart of water, and during the day, the decoction is to be drank, and the leaves eaten.

No. 87.—ANOTHER FOR THE SAME.

Take a gallon of fresh strong beer about milk warm, and mix a handful of horse-radish bruised, a handful of fennel roots bruised, a handful of parsley roots, and tops, a handful of burdock roots, a handful of the bark of the roots of elder, a handful of spice wood, a handful of water cresses, a handful of sarsaparilla, all to be bruised and put into the beer, with a sufficient quantity of yeast to work it. Let it stand for twenty-four hours, then strain it, and it will be fit for use.

No. 88.—ANOTHER FOR THE SAME.

Take two large handfuls of fern, scrape it a little to take off the dirt, and put it to boil in a large pitcher full of water during two hours. It is used at meals like other water. You must make use of the fern that has but one branch, because the sort that has many branches is not proper.

No. 89.—FOR THE SAME.

Almost all persons afflicted with the dropsy, are cured by taking through their mouth or in glyster, every third day, a decoction of worm-wood, and polypody.

No. 90.—PTISAN OR TEA, FOR THE DROPSY.

Take some root of large nettles, that are yellow, with some marrow of elder, one handful of dandelion leaves, and dog's grass root, boil the whole in three quarts of water, until reduced to two quarts, and let the patient drink one glass of it every morning fasting. At his meals, some may be mixed with wine, and must drink of it, as often as he is thirsty.

No. 91.—FOR THE SAME.

Take one large handful of parsley, wild succory roots, and fennel roots, and one handful of sage. You must pick out the strings or cords that are in the roots, and boil the whole in eight quarts of spring water in a new glazed pot, and let it consume to one half, then strain it through a linen cloth, a put up this water into phials well stopped. The patient must take, fasting, one glass of it, into which glass you must have put two fingers breadth of good white wine, that it be neither sweet nor tart, and the patient must not eat for three hours after; the same dose must be repeated three hours after dinner, and the same regimen observed and continued until a cure takes place.

No. 92.—FOR THE SAME.

Take some charvil, pound it, then soak the juice and the herb in a gill of wine during one night; then strain it and give it to the patient. This is likewise a sovereign remedy for the cure of the dropsy.

No. 93.—FOR THE SAME.

Three scruples of loadstone powder, taken with fennel juice, does securely cure the dropsy.

Glysters made of the decoction of thistle with urine, cure the dropsy, if that remedy be often repeated. Here follows another remedy well proved: take lard and wolfs liver one drachm and a half of each, they being pounded, mix them with syrup of sea wormwood, and make of the whole eighteen pills; the patient afflicted with the dropsy must take three of them, in the morning fasting, and he will happily recover.

No. 94.—FOR THE CURE OF THE EPILEPSY.

Take some of the after birth of a woman, wash and pound it well, after mix it with rye flour, in order to make bread with it, and bake it in an oven, the patient must take the weight of half an ounce of it, to eat, morning and evening, every first day of the first quarter of the moon.

The most part of the remedies that have been given for the apoplexy, may also be used in this case; therefore, they may be resorted to when necessary.

No. 95.—AGAINST THE SAME.

As soon as a child is born, and before it takes anything else, if you make it swallow half a scruple of coral in powder, it is given for certain, that the child will never be afflicted with the Epilepsy.

No. 96.—FOR THE SAME.

Take some wheat flour, that you will mix with dew, make of it a cake, which being baked, give it to the patient and he will get well.

No. 97.—ANOTHER FOR THE SAME.

If you cut and open the young ones of the swallows of the first next; you will find in their ventricle, two small stones, one of which is all of one color, and the other of several colors; before they touch ground, shut them up in a piece of goat or deerskin, and tie them on the arm and neck: they will cure the patient of the Epilepsy.

No. 98.—FOR SORE EYES.

Pour into a large long necked bottle, one pint of water of roses, fennel water and euphrasia water, of each two ounces, thirty grains of cloves, the same quantity of rosemary flowers, half an ounce of sugar candy, conserve of roses; a pinch of provins roses. Stop your vessel well, put it to digest five or six days, and expose it to the sun from the month of June to the month of August; after which strain the liquor through a white linen cloth, without pressing it, and keep it in a glass vessel well corked. Make use of it in the disease mentioned above, in rubbing with it the afflicted part, and applying over it a linen cloth dipped in this water.

No. 99.—FOR THE FLUX.

Mix vinegar and salt together, and drink a small quantity of it frequently, which will be an immediate and effectual cure. I had opportunities of seeing this cure tried, and never knew it to fail. I have even known it to cure those whose bowels physicians had declared to be mortified.

No. 100.—FOR THE BLOODY FLUX OR LOOSENESS OF THE BOWELS.

Take the juice of elder berries, when it is well ripe; pass them through a cloth or searge, in order the better to clean it, afterwards take some good wheat flour, as much as you think proper, and make use of that juice instead of water, to make of them some small loaves, which you will put in an oven with other bread to bake, taking care that they do not burn; owing to their small size: if they are not dry at the first baking, they must be put in the oven a second time, in order that they become as dry within as without, to be put in powder: afterwards, make of them some small packages, or papers, after having passed it through a fine seive. The dose and quantity to be given, is the weight of one ounce for grown persons; and for children the fourth part of that dose, say a quarter of an ounce.

No. 101.—FOR BLOODY FLUX AND LOOSENESS.

Take one gill of water of roses, infuse in it two ounces of roses of provins, during twelve hours, on some warm ashes, then strain it and put into it the weight of one ounce of rhubarb, cut in small pieces, infuse the whole twelve hours longer, then having strained and pressed it, put in a skillet over the fire, with two ounces of sugar, to make a syrup.

The patient must, on the first day, take two spoonfuls of it, fasting, and one spoonful every day, he must be one hour and a half after taking the dose, without eating, and continue the same treatment until the complaint ceases; this remedy is infallible.

No. 102.—FOR BLOODY FLUX ONLY.

You must take in the morning, in an egg, cooked in the usual way, half a spoonful of a small seed of the silverweed, (a plant) that is usually found amongst seedsmen, after having well stirred and mixed it with the egg, and repeat the same two or three times; this performs wonders in a very short time.

No. 103.—FOR LOOSENESS AND BLOOD FLUX.

Take some dock seed, (a sort of sorrel) that grows amongst the wheat, pound it, and put it in some broth: this is one of the most sovereign remedies.

No. 104.—FOR THE SAME AT ALL TIMES.

Take a new laid egg, and beat well together the yellow and white; then with some wheat flour, make a kind of a cake, and while you are making the dough, grate a nutmeg amongst it: the dough being well made, and the whole well worked and stirred, bake this cake between ashes, then give it hot just out of the fire, to the patient, he must while eating it, drink two or three times, either wine or gin.

No. 105.—FOR A LOOSENESS IN THE BOWELS.

Take some pounded panic, (a sort of corn,) and give it to the patient to drink with wine, and he will recover. The same panic, being boiled with goat's milk, and eat twice a day, morning and evening, will operate the same.

No. 106.—FOR THE SAME.

Take some green horse beans, with their shells on, boil them with vinegar; eat them so with their shells, and the looseness will stop.

No. 107.—FOR THE SAME.

Take some green oak acorn, bruise them well with their shells, and by the means of a still, draw some water from it, of which you will give to the patient: this remedy is very salutary.

The remedies that have been already described for the dysentery and looseness can likewise be used.

No. 108.—TO STRENGTHEN THE LEGS AND FEET.

To make fomentations for the legs, thighs, and feet, make a decoction of sage, rosemary, thyme, lavender, cammomile flowers, and melilot, stewed in white or red wine; or else make some lye with oak leaves, a little vinegar, and half a handful of salt.

This decoction has the virtue to subtilize, attenuate, cut, resolve, dissipate, and dry up the gross and viscous humours.

No. 109.—FOR THE GOUT.

Take snake headed irs, scammony, white turbith, liquorice, cinnamon, half a drachm of each; of the ingredients more or less, but always in equal quantity. Reduce the whole to powder, and pass it through a fine seive. The patient must take the weight of half an ounce, or one fourth less, that will depend on the difficulty he has of being purged. This powder must be soaked in the evening in half a glass of white wine, and on the following morning, mix the whole well, and let the patient take it, two hours after a broth. He must keep his room.

No. 110.—FOR THE SAME.

Press some green olives before they are ripe, and extract the oil, which must be kept in a bottle, into which you put some henbane leaves, so that the oil covers them a great deal; and the whole must be kept well shut up. This oil is excellent at the end of two months, it must be applied lukewarm over the part afflicted with pains; and it will appease them. It moreover prevents a pain, if it be applied when there is none.

No. 111.—PLASTER FOR THE GOUT.

Oil of roses one drachm, Burgundy pitch, and black pitch, two drachms of each; saffron two scruples; opium dissolved in cow's milk, three scruples; pepper, one drachm; and make of all these things a plaster in the usual way.

No. 112.—CATAPLASM FOR GOUT.

Take some crumbs of wheat bread, and goat's milk, eight ounces of each, house leek juice, one ounce, the yolks of three eggs, and half a drachm of saffron; make of the whole a cataplasm, and make use of it.

No. 113.—AGAINST THE GONORRHEA.

Take an equal quantity of sorrel, renufar, running thistles and strawberry roots; make a ptisan, or a tea of them.

No. 114.—FOR INFLAMMATION OF THE REINS.

Take oil of roses, one drachm, white wax washed with rose water, and melted, two drachms; mix the whole together, and make an ointment of it, which you make use of in anointing the region of the reins.

No. 115.—FOR INDIGESTION AND LUBRICITY OF THE BOWELS.

Take one ounce of dried orange peel, fine powdered; divide it into scruples, and take one scruple at a time, drink a glass of wine after it. This is a medicine not disgusting, not costly, easily tried, and if not found useful, easily left off. Do not take too much in haste; a scruple once in three hours, or about five scruples a day, will be sufficient to begin, or less, if you find any aversion. Best without sugar; if syrup, old syrup of quinces, but even that I do not like; I think better of conserve of sloes.

No. 116.—FOR JAUNDICE.

Cook a whole lime, under hot ashes; then cut it, and put it to soak in white wine; which the patient must drink in the morning fasting.

No. 117.—FOR THE JAUNDICE ON THE FACE, PROCEEDING FROM THE OVERFLOWING OF THE GALL.

Take a large white onion, in which you will make a hole on the germ, in throwing the green part away; put in that hole, the size of a chestnut of good treacle, bake it slowly before the fire, but take care it is not burnt or roasted, or get dirty amongst the ashes. When it will be done, put it in a white linen, and press well the juice out of it; the patient must drink it in the morning, fasting, and during twenty days. The jaundice and paleness will disappear.

No. 118.—FOR THE YELLOW JAUNDICE.

Parch Indian corn, and eat freely of it; I have know this to cure when no other medicine would; I am a witness of three who have been perfectly cured by making use of the above.

No. 119.—FOR THE SAME.

Take a large handful of the bark of the black alder, scraped or cut small, boil it in a quart of sound hard cider; let the patient drink freely of it when cold.

No. 120.—FOR THE LOCK JAW.

Dip the part afflicted in a quantity of warm lye, as strong as possible; but if it be a part of the body, which cannot be immersed, rub the part afflicted with a flannel soaked in the lye. This has never failed in one instance.

No. 121.—TO REPAIR THE LIVER WHEN UNPURE.

Take one handful of smeallage, the same quantity of sage, and colt's foot, pound it well, afterwards, put into it one quart of white wine, then strain the whole through a cloth. Let the patient take of it during three days, on the morning, fasting; and let him not eat for two hours after.

No. 122.—AGAINST DEAFNESS.

The juice of cabbage, dropped in the ear, affords a wonderful relief against deafness, that may come through causes of sickness.

No. 123.—FOR BRUISED NERVES.

Take some deer marrow, and melt it with French brandy, then rub the painful parts with it.

No. 124.—AN OINTMENT FOR NEW SORES.

Take half a pound of Venice turpentine, laurel oil, one drachm sage juice, two drachms, gum elemi, half a drachm; with which make an ointment.

No. 125.—AN OINTMENT FOR SORES AND PRICKINGS.

Turpentine of Venice, two drachms, white wax and oil of roses, two scruples of each, bethony juice, half a pound; of the whole, make an ointment secundum artem.

No. 126.—AN OINTMENT FOR FALLS, WOUNDS, CONTUSIONS, CUTS, &c.

Take four pounds of mice dung, pound them, and put them in a new pot glazed inside, add to it one pound of fresh butter; boil the whole during a short time, and strain it through a linen, and in this liquid, put two ounces of turpentine, and finish boiling the whole. This is a wonderful ointment.

No. 127.—FOR PALSY.

Make a decoction of apex, one ounce of it, and boil it a little longer than one quarter of an hour; the patient must take a glass of it before meals. This remedy must be continued one year before it can perform a perfect cure.

No. 128.—FOR THE SAME.

Take a young kid, dress it, stuff its belly with one pound of cloves, roast it on the spit, and with the grease that will come out, rub the afflicted part. Instead of a kid, take a very fat duck, and prepare it in the same manner as mentioned above for the kid. This remedy is well approved.

No. 129.—FOR THE PLEURISY.

The remedy for this disease is easy. A cataplasm made with dregs of wine, must be put on paper as hot as the patient can bear it on the afflicted part. This affords a wonderful relief, which is followed with a general perspiration, and a cure will in a short time take place.

No. 130.—FOR THE SAME.

This remedy is not less efficacious than that which we have just given, it consists in making a cold infusion, during three or four hours, in a gill of white wine, some fresh and yet warm balls of horse dung, after having broken them in pieces. The wine is afterwards strained, and given to the patient, who will not fail to get cured, through perspiration.

No. 131.—FOR THE INFLAMMATION OF THE LUNGS AND SPLEEN.

The patient must constantly drink of a tea made with speekwell; a little sugar must be added to it. The patient must not be bled. This potion or tea provokes the urine.

Or else, make a tea with viper's grass, and let the patient drink constantly of it. This tea causes a great perspiration and the spitting of the abscess, should there be any in the breast. This remedy is also good for the small pox.

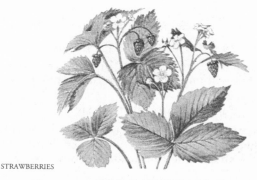

STRAWBERRIES

No. 133.—FOR PAINS IN THE BREAST

Take one pint of water, put it into a pan or kettle, and add to it one handful of wheat bran with the size of an egg of fine sugar; let the whole together take one boiling; then strain it, and let the patient drink this water as hot as he can bear it. This remedy must be repeated several times a day.

No. 134.—FOR A WEAK BREAST AND LUNGS.

Make often use of damas raisins, boiled in wine during one quarter of an hour, and in a short time your breast will recover its strength.

No. 135.—CABBAGE SYRUP FOR THE BREAST AND LUNGS.

Take some cabbages, and pound them with their leaves and stalks, strain it, and add the same weight of very good honey. Boil the whole together, and scum it continually, and when it does not scum any more, the syrup will be done. One spoonful of it is sufficient to be taken, fasting.

No. 136.—TO EXTIRPATE WARTS.

Take an equal quantity of brown soap, and spittle; mix the whole together, and make a plaster of it; apply it on the warts and leave it on them twenty-four hours; then take it off, and at the same time, the warts and roots will come off.

No. 137.—FOR WARTS ON THE HANDS.

Pound some horseradish roots, and wash the warts with it two or three times a day.

No. 138.—TO CAUSE THE WARTS, IN WHATEVER PART THEY BE, TO FALL OFF.

Take a sheep lung, newly killed, let the blood drain off from it, and as soon as there is no more blood on it, press the lung in a press, some water will come out; keep this water in a glass bottle and rub the warts with, and they will disappear.

No. 139.—TO PURGE THE BRAIN.

Take some goats milk, and draw it in through your nose, three or four times; this will entirely remove from the brain all obstruction.

No. 140.—FOR HEADACHE.

The water that comes out of walnut tree, after an incision has been made in them, the quantity of one ounce drank at intervals, appeases in a short time the headache, however violent.

No. 141.—FOR BLEEDING AT THE NOSE.

Put one drop of vinegar in the ear of the person whose nose is bleeding, on the side of the nostril through which the blood comes out. This will stop it.

No. 142.—FOR LOSS OF BLOOD IN WOMEN.

Take some pervinca, let it get dry, and reduce it to powder. The patient must take the weight of half an ounce of it, with some broth, fasting.

No. 143.—PLASTER AGAINST HARDNESS OF BREASTS.

It is made with horse beans meal, and barley meal, half an ounce of each, flax-seed and sangreen meals, six drachms of each, and one scruple of saffron.

No. 144.—FOR TUMORS AND INFLAMMATIONS OF THE BREASTS.

Take a small handful of plantain and mallow leaves, boil them in a sufficient quantity of rose water until it is consumed to a thickness, afterwards, add to it two ounces of barley flour, one ounce and a half of oil of roses, of the whole form a plaster.

No. 145.—FOR SWELLINGS, ARISING FROM DROPSY OR OTHER CAUSES.

You must have a great quantity of elder bark, boil them with three quarts of white wine, until they are reduced to two quarts; afterwards strain and press them hard, and drink of it morning and evening.

No. 146.—PLASTER FOR A SWELLING IN THE KNEES.

Take some cow dung, and vinegar, mix them together and boil them until some thickness; then apply this plaster on the afflicted part; the swelling will soon disappear, as it has often been experienced.

No. 147.—FOR SWELLINGS THAT CAUSE PAIN.

Take the crumbs of rye bread, and some vinegar, boil them together, and apply it warm on the sick part, and the pain will cease.

No. 148.—FOR THE SAME.

Boil some flaxseed with ewes milk, and apply it often and warm, on the swelling.

No. 149.—AGAINST RHEUMATISM.

You must boil on the fire a glass of the urine of the person afflicted with it, then, bathe the afflicted part; afterwards, dip a linen folded double in the urine, apply it on the pain and tie it up. This remedy consumes and dissipates the humours entirely.

No. 150.—FOR THE SAME.

The afflicted part must be rubbed before the fire with a linen, and take some elder oil, in which five or six drops of spirits of wine have been mixed, rub with it the pain every morning and evening with a greasy towel, and applied on the painful part, when the patient is going to bed.

No. 151.—FOR SCALDS AND BURNS.

As soon as the accident has happened, take a plaster of tar, the size of the wound, and apply it to the place affected. By this simple application, which has been often tried and never found wanting, the inflammation will be found to subside, and the pain to cease in a few minutes.

No. 152.—FOR SORE THROAT.

Take some rye flour, boil it in a pint of milk, during half a quarter of an hour, then take two lily onions, and make a cataplasm of it, which must be applied lukewarm about the throat: it causes a wonderful effect.

No. 153.—TO DISSOLVE THE APOSTHUMES AND ABSCESSES THAT COME ABOUT THE THROAT.

You must have some dry ass dung, and swallow dung, put them in powder, which you will mix with warm water. The patient must very often make use of it as a gargle. This remedy is very certain.

No. 154.—FOR FALLEN PALATE.

If through a great distillation of humours or fluxions, the palate is fallen; cabbage juice applied on the head, has the virtue to draw it up and put it again in its place.

No. 155.—FOR THE TREMBLING OF THE HANDS.

Mugwort soaked in water, is very useful to strengthen trembling hands, by washing them often with it.

No. 156.—AGAINST VAPOURS AND HEADACHE.

Bathing the legs with lukewarm water, grapevine leaves, appeases in a short time the vapours, and the headache.

No. 157.—COMPOSITION OF THE VENEREAL POWDER.

Take senna in powder, lignumvitae, sarsaparilla, two scruples of each; cinnamon and aniseed, one scruple of each. The dose to be taken is one drachm infused in some white wine during the night, and drink it in the morning with the powder.

No. 158.—FOR SWELLED TESTICLES.

Take some rue, and having pounded it, apply it on the parts, and the swelling will immediately disappear.

No. 159.—FOR TUMOURS IN TESTICLES.

You must have four ounces of the four following kinds of flour, to wit; barley, rye, flax and ervum, boil the whole with beer: that being done, add to it one ounce of camomile oil, roses, camomile and melliot one drachm of each. Of the whole make a cataplasm to be applied on the sick parts.

No. 160.—FOR THE SAME.

Nothing is better for worms in children, than the worms themselves dried on a red hot tile, and reduced to powder. Give this powder to the sick children, and it will expel all those with which they are troubled.

No. 161.—WINE AGAINST WORMS, CUTTING PAINS AND LOOSENESS IN THE BOWELS.

Take twenty pomegranates, after they are pounded put them in a vessel with some thick wine. Then stop up the vessel, and do not open it but at the end of thirty days: after which time, take some of this liquor fasting, and you will be free from all those diseases or indispositions.

No. 162.—FOR ULCERS IN THE MOUTH.

You must take some honeysuckle leaves and distill them. Make use of the water to gargle the ulcers in your mouth and throat with it, and they will infallibly get cured.

No. 163.—AGAINST THE FLUX AND URINE.

You must have some tender points of oak leaves, and boil them in wine; then pound them, make a cataplasm, and apply it on the patient's privy member, and he will in a short time be cured.

No. 164.—WATER FOR HAND WORMS.

Make a lye with flaxseed; with which you must wash your hands during eight days.

Mint juice is also very excellent, in rubbing your hand with it.

No. 165.—WATER FOR ULCERS AND SORES.

Take one ounce of long aristolochy, put it in powder or only bruised; four ounces of common sugar, one quart of white wine; boil the whole in an earthen glazed pot, until the consummation of half a pint upon the whole; then strain it and keep this water for use when necessary.

No. 166.—WATER TO TAKE THE REDNESS, ITCHING AND BLEAREDNESS OF THE EYES.

Take two ounces of water of roses, the same quantity of white wine; mix together, and rub the eyes with it.

No. 167.—FOR REDNESS AND WEAKNESS IN THE EYES.

Apply on the afflicted eyes, in form of a small cataplasm, some single daisies, withered on a hot shovel, and bruised, before they are applied to the eyes.

No. 168.—AGAINST THE FEVERS OF CHILDREN.

It will not be found less strange, which has been tried several times, that by putting a large cucumber near a child at the breast, having a fever, when the child is asleep, the fever will leave him without fail.

No. 169.—FOR DEAFNESS AND DIZZINESS.

Peal Garlic, dip it in honey, and put it into the ear, with a little black wool. Lie with that ear uppermost, and put the same into the other ear the next night. Do this, if necessary, for eight or ten nights.

No. 170.—FOR GRAVEL OR STONE.

Take lobelia, violets, and rib wort, of each a handful. To this, add one pint of white lie, and boil the composition ten or twelve minutes; then strain off the decoction, and add one pint of Holland gin. Take as much as the stomach will bear, six times a day. At the same time, take a glass of the juice of onion tops every night.

No. 171.—ANOTHER.

Take two pounds of hard root, called ox balm; two pounds of queen of the meadow, called by the Indians, Sofia; two pounds of ginsang root, with the roots washed clean and cut them fine. Then boil them half a day with clear water, in a tight covered pot. You must not skim, strain, or suffer it to boil over, nor let it remain in an iron vessel over night.

This compound is for two quarts. When this syrup is settled, drain it off, and add a pint of Holland gin, and a pound of loaf sugar. Take this syrup as hot as it can be drank, as much, and as often as the constitution will admit, until the gravel or stone is dissolved. This will be found a stone dissolving application, and should it cut or dissolve the stone or gravel so fast as to clog the neck of the bladder, as is often the case, the patient must take diuretic syrup.

No. 172.—ANOTHER.

Make a strong tea of the herb called heart's ease, and Jacob's ladder, and make a very strong tea, drink plentifully of it, and it is a most certain remedy.

No. 173.—ANOTHER.

Infuse one ounce of wild parsley seed in a pint of white wine, for twelve days.—Drink a glass before breakfast, fasting, for three months, and breakfast for three months on agrimony tea.

No. 174.—ANOTHER.

Pour hot water to a good handful of gravel weed, and as soon as the strength is drawn out, give the patient two gills; and in an hour give another, and so on till it begins to operate. Then once in two hours, and as the gravel begins to come away, in three hours, then once in six and so continue until well. This I consider the most sovereign remedy, that has ever been found out.

No. 175.—FOR BILIOUS COMPLAINTS.

Take the leaves of tobacco, boil them in pure water until very strong. To one quart of this liquor, add three gills of rum, and three gills of sale molasses; then bottle it up, and take as much of this as the stomach will bear, once a day. This wholly prevents the billious cholic.

No. 176.—FOR ASTHMA.

Put two teaspoonsful of pulverized lobelia into a pint of rum, and use it for a bitter morning and evening. Half a gill will be sufficient at once.

No. 177.—ANOTHER.

Take two ounces of spignard root, two ounces of sweet flag root, two ounces elecampane. Beat them fine in a mortar, and add a pound of honey, beat well together. A teaspoonful is a dose, three times a day.

No. 178.—ANOTHER.

Take lobelia, blood root, the roots of blue violets, of each a teaspoonful when pulverized. Boil them fifteen minutes in six gills of water. Strain out the powders, and add to the decoction, an equal quantity of good rum, and take six times a day, sufficient to nauciate or make sick at the stomach, but not puke.

After taking the above, make a syrup of garden celendine, dogmachy bark, hog brake, and white Solomon's seal root. Make a syrup of this by boiling a handful of each in twelve quarts of water down to one; then add spirits and honey, and it is fit for use. Take two glasses a day, fasting; that is, two hours before breakfast or supper.

No. 179.—ANOTHER.

Beat saffron blows, fine, and take eight or ten grains every night, on sliced apples.

No. 180.—FOR SPITTING BLOOD.

Take two spoonsful of nettles every morning, and a large teacupful of the decoction of nettles at night, for a week. This presently stops either spitting or vomiting blood; or half a teaspoonful of Barbadoes tar, or a lump of sugar at night. It most commonly effects a cure at once.

No. 181.—ANOTHER.

Take a pound of yellow dock root, dry it thoroughly, pound it
fine, boil it in a quart of sweet milk, strain it off, and drink a gill
three times a day, or pound balm of Gilead buds with brown sugar, to that degree that you can make them into pills. Take four
or five of these at going to bed, and it wonderfully helps the
soreness in the stomach.

No. 182.—POULTICE FOR OLD SORES.

Scrape carrots, with them on a fire shovel, until very soft; apply it to the sore and it takes out the inflammation. It is an excellent poultice for sore breasts; and perhaps there is nothing better that can be applied to the eyes that are sore and inflamed.

No. 183.—FOR AN ESSENCE.

This is an excellent essence, and good for all sorts of inward
weakness, pain in the side, stomach or breast, coughs &c.—Take
twenty pounds of fir boughs, one pound of spignard, and
three pounds of red clover. Put them into a still with ten gallons
of cider; then draw off three gallons, and drink half a glass night
and morning.

No. 184.—FOR INWARD PILES.

Swallow a pill of pitch fasting. One pill generally cures the
first trial.

No. 185.—FOR BLEEDING PILES.

Lightly boil the juice of nettles with a little sugar, and take two
ounces. It needs repeating.

No. 186.—FOR AGUE.

Take a handful of hops, boil them in a pint of water, and drink
of this decoction just before the cold fit comes on. It will stop the
fit for this time, if not throw it off. Proceed in this way a few
times, and it will effect a cure.

No. 187.—FOR SALT RHEUM.

First, cleanse the blood by making a decoction of dogmachy
bark, and ground hemlock, (not cicuta). Add one pint of gin to a
quart of this decoction, and take a glass three times a day. After
taking this one week, make an ointment by simmering six common frogs in one pound of hog's lard or fresh butter, two hours.
With this ointment frequently anoint the part affected.

No. 188.—ANOTHER.

Take blue flag root, river willow, the bark of the root, boiled in pure water very strong. Strain and add hog's lard, and continue boiling until the water is all evaporated, and when cold it is fit for use. Anoint the parts affected, twice a day, until well.—It also cures the piles.

Steep the root of cockawash jammed up in cold water, six or eight hours; then wash the parts affected, with the decoction three or four times a day, and drink two glasses a day of this steeped in another vessel for that purpose. It is a certain cure.

No. 189.—FOR SORE NIPPLES.

When the infant stops sucking, apply a plaster of the balsam of fir, and it will cure in four days.

No. 190.—FOR ITCHING HEELS.

Take tallow and rub the part affected with it; rub it in by a hot fire at night going to bed, and repeat it three or four times. A certain cure.

No. 191.—FOR BLOODSHOT EYES.

Apply boiled hysop and rue, as a poultice. This is a sure remedy, as frequently proved.

No. 192.—FOR CLOUDED EYES.

Take a drachm of powdered Bethony every morning in milk. This is infallible.

No. 193.—FOR DULL SIGHT.

Steep the bag wherein the musk of a skunk is contained, in half a gill of water. Dip a soft rag in the water gently daub the eyes two or three times a day.

No. 194.—FOR FILMS ON THE EYE.

Mix the juice of ground Ivy, that is, gill-go-by-the-ground, with a little honey. Drop it in morning and evening.

No. 195.—FOR HUMOURS IN THE EYES.

Apply a few drops of refined sugar, melted in brandy, to the eye; or boil a handful of bramble brier leaves, in one quart of spring water to a pint. Drop this frequently into the eye. This also cures cankers or any sores.

No. 196.—FOR INFLAMED EYES.

Apply as a poultice, boiled roasted or rotten apples, warm; and this will hardly fail; or wormwood tops, with the yolk of an egg. This is a fine remedy.

No. 197.—ANOTHER.

Stamp and strain ground ivy, and daisies, an equal quantity. Add a little rose water and loaf sugar, and drop a drop or two at a time in the eye, and it takes away all manner of inflammation, smarting, itching, spots, webs, or any other disorder.

No. 198.—FOR FROZEN LIMBS.

Plunge them into cold water until the frost is out, and then anoint them with grease.

No. 199.—FOR UVULA RELAXED.

Bruise a cabbage leaf, and lay it on hot, on the crown of the head. Repeat it if necessary, in two hours. I never knew it to fail.

No. 200.—FOR THE BLOODY FLUX.

Take a puke of mullen leaves pounded, add to them a little water on the leaves, press out the juice, clarify it by scalding it over the fire then add to it a quart of brandy, and let the patient drink a tablespoonful every hour.

No. 201.—ANOTHER.

Or take blood weed called horse tail, and comfrey roots, boiled together, sweetened with honey, and drink often of it.

No. 202.—ANOTHER.

Or take sweet flag root, boiled in milk, and sweetened with honey.—Drink often of this medicine, taking a gill at a time.

Drink often of a tea made of white pine bark, spikenard and everlasting.

No. 203.—FOR PALSY OF THE HANDS.

Wash them often in a decoction of sage, as hot as you can bear. I know of nothing better; or two or three spoonsful of mustard seed in a quart of water, and wash often in this as hot as may be.

No. 204.—FOR PALPITATION OF THE HEART.

Take the saw dust made from a pitch pine knot, the tops of vervine and agrimony, of each a handful, pulverize the herbs, and put them into two quarts of wine, let them infuse twelve hours, and it is fit for use. Take a small glass three times a day, and it seldom fails.

BOTANIC GARDEN.

GARDEN CELENDINE; PILE WORT; OR FIG WORT.

1. The virtues of this herb are known by experience, that the decoction of the leaves and roots, doth most wonderfully help the piles and hemorrhoids; as also, kernels by the ears and throat, called kings evil, or any other hard wens or tumors. Celendine, made into an oil, ointment or plaster readily cures the piles, hemorrhoids or kings evil. The very herb borne around the body next the skin, helps in such diseases, though it never touch the place aggrieved. With this I cured a lady of the kings evil, broke the sore, drew out a gill of corrupted matter and cured it without any scar in one week.

CINQUEFOIL; OR FIVE FINGERS.

2. This spreads and crawls far upon the ground, with long slender strings like strawberries, which take root again and shoot forth many leaves made of five parts dented about the edges, and somewhat hard. The stalks are slender, leaning downwards and bear many small yellow flowers with some yellow threads in the middle, standing about a small and green edge; which, when it is ripe, is a little rough, and contains small brown seeds. The root is of a blackish brown colour, seldom so large as one's little finger but grows long with some threads attached to it. It grows by wood and path ways on piles, and in almost every place. This herb has great virtues. If you give twenty grains of the powdered herb in wine or wine vinegar, it will seldom miss curing an ague of whatever nature or kind. The juice thereof drank, about four ounces at a time for certain days, cures the quinsy and yellow jaundice, and taken for thirty days cures the falling sickness.—The roots boiled in milk and drank, is a most effectual remedy for all fluxes either in men or women. A decoction of the root boiled in vinegar, eases the toothache. The juice and a little honey helps the hoarseness of the throat, and is very good for a cough.—The root boiled in vinegar helps all knots, kernels, hard swellings and inflammations and St. Anthony's fire.

COMFREY.

3. This is a well known garden herb, it is good against all inward hurts, bruises and wounds: that is, the decoction drank, cureth the same. It is good for women that have immoderate courses, and a syrup of the root is effectual in all these complaints. The root being pounded and applied outwardly, is good for wounds, ruptures, broken bones, knotted breasts, hemorrhoids, inflammations, gout, pained joints, gangrenes.

YELLOW DAISY, OR CROW FOOT.

4. This herb grows in abundance in our country, on meadow or pasture grounds. It grows from one to two feet high, has a roundish leaf and blows in the forepart of summer—the blows are of a bright yellow colour. The herb, if bruised and applied to the skin, draws as perfect a blister as the Spanish fly: but the better way is to mix it with salve. The juice is good on application to palsied limbs and cold swellings: it stimulates and produces a degree of excitement.

WAKE ROBIN, MARCH TURNIP; OR CUCKOO POINT.

5. This herb, if a teaspoonful of the powdered root be given, is a present sure remedy for poison and plague. A little vinegar with it allays the biting taste upon the tongue. The said powder taken in wine as other drink, procures urine and brings down women's courses, and purges them effectually after child bearing; taken with sheeps milk, it heals inward ulcers. The leaves either green or dry, or the juice of them will cleanse all manner of rotten and filthy ulcers in any part of the body. The decoction of the root dropped into the eyes, cleanses them from any film or skin, clouds or mists that begin to hinder the sight. The juice dropped into the ear eases the pain of earache.

DANDELION.

6. This herb is well known and grows frequently in all meadows and pasture grounds, and is of an opening and cleansing quality and therefore very effectually opens obstructions of the liver and gall. It wonderfully opens the passages of the urine both in old and young; it powerfully cleanses imposthumes and inward ulcers. The decoction of the roots or leaves in white wine, or leaves boiled as pot herbs, is very effectual. It is good for a person drawing towards a consumption, and many times will produce a healthful state.

DOVE'S FOOT OR, CRANE'S BILL.

7. This herb has divers small, round, pale green leaves, cut in about the edges much like mallows, standing upon long reddish hairy stalks, lying in a round compass upon the ground. It has very small bright, red flowers, of five leaves a piece, when they seed they form short beaks or bills.

The herb is very good for the wind cholic, as also to expel the stone and gravel in the kidneys. The decoction is good for inward wounds and bruises and to stay the bleeding thereof, and will expel congealed blood. The decoction in wine is a good foment to ease the pain of the gout. It is of singular use for ruptures and bursts in either old or young.

ELECAMPANE.

8. This herb needs no description. The fresh roots of elecampane preserved in sugar, or made into syrup is very effectual to warm a cold windy stomach, and to help the cough, shortness of breath, wheezing of the lungs. The dried root powdered and mixed with sugar, answers the same purpose, and is good for a stoppage in the urine, or of women's courses. The root and herb, beaten and made into beer and drank daily, strengthens the sight of the eyes wonderfully.—The decoction of the roots in wine, drives forth and kills all manner of worms that people are troubled with. It is good to fasten loose teeth, spitting blood, cramps, gout, cankers, &c.

EYE BRIGHT.

9. Eye bright is generally known. If this herb was but as much used as it is neglected, it would half spoil the spectacle maker's trade. The juice, distilled water, or decoction of eye bright dropped into the eyes for a number of days, helps all inflammation of the eyes and dimness of sight; almost any way prepared, it is a powerful remedy for weak sore eyes, and to strengthen those that are dim through age.

FEATHERFEW.

10. This is an excellent herb to open obstructions of the body, and a great strengthener of women, and will remedy such infirmities as a careless midwife has been the cause of; in such cases it will do them all the good they can wish for. A decoction of the herb made in wine or of the flowers, or a syrup, or apply the boiled herb outwardly to the parts, does wonderfully help. It is good against the gravel, to cleanse away phlegm to cure melancholy, headache, ague cholic.

FENNEL.

11. Fennel is good against wind in the stomach; is useful to increase milk in women's breasts and make it wholesome for the child, also to prevent sickness in the stomach, shortness of breath and wheezing; to open obstructions of the liver, and to cause urine. The seeds and roots are much used in drinks and broths to make people more spare and lean that are too fat.

WINTER GREEN.

12. This is a singular good herb, and especially to heal green wounds. A salve made of the green herbs stamped, or the juice boiled, with hogs lard or with sallad oil and wax, and some turpentine added to it, is sovereign salve, and highly extolled by the Germans, who affirm it to heal all manner of wounds. A decoction of the herb, or in wine, and given to drink, does wonderfully help ulcers, fluxes, women's courses, bleeding of wounds, inflammations rising upon pains of the heart, cankers or fistulas, and the distilled waters answer the same purpose.

ARTICHOKES.

13. The decoction of the juice of artichokes, is good to open the passages of the urine, and of course is good for stone in the bladder.

HEMP.

14. This herb is good for something else besides making halters of. The seed steeped, is excellent for wind in the stomach; it opens obstructions of the gall, and is good against all fluxes, and is very good to kill the worms either in man or beast. The juice dropped into the ears, kills the worms in them, and draws forth ear wigs. A decoction of the root is good to allay inflammation in the head or any other part, or pains of the gout, joints, shrinking of sinews, pains of the hips.

HYSOP.

15. Hysop is known to be a garden herb. Hysop boiled with rew and honey, helps cough, shortness of breath, and wheezing, and rheumatic complaints. It helps to destroy worms in children, and being taken with figs and nitre, helps the dropsy. Being boiled with wine, it is good to wash inflammations; and takes away the black and blue spots that come by bruises, or falls; it is an excellent remedy for the quinsy, or swellings in the throat; it helps the toothache, being boiled in vinegar, and gargled therewith, the hot vapour of the decoction conveyed into the ear, eases the inflammation and singing noise of them. The oil of it kills lice, and helps the itching of the head. The green herb bruised with a little vinegar does quickly heal any cut or wound.

JUNIPER BUSH.

16. The juniper berries are a most admirable counter poison, and as great a resister of the pestilence as any that grows. They are excellent against the bitings of venomous beasts; they cause urine; it is a powerful remedy against the dropsy, even if the ashes of the bush be made into lye and drank, cures the disease. —It provokes the terms in women, helps the fits of the mother, strengthens the stomach exceedingly, and expels wind. Indeed there is scarce a better remedy for wind than the chymical oil drawn from the berries. Those that know not how to extract the oil, may eat ten or twelve of the berries each morning, fasting. They are admirably good for a cough, shortness of breath and consumption, pains in the bowels, ruptures, cramps, and convulsions. They give speedy and safe delivery to women with child. The ashes of the wood made into lye, cures the itch, scabs, and leprosy. The berries break the stone, procure appetite that is lost.

HOPS.

17. Hops are so well known that they need no description. Every good housewife is acquainted with them. The decoction of the hops is good to open obstructions of the liver and spleen, to cleanse the blood, and help costiveness; is good against the gravel. They help to cure the French disease, and all manner of scabs, itch, and other breakings out of the body; as also tetters, ringworms and spreading sores. Half a drachm of the seed in powder taken in drink, kills worms in the body, helps the terms in women, eases the headaches which arises from heat. A syrup made of the juice and sugar, cures the yellow jaundice, tempers the heat of the stomach and liver.

HORSETAIL.

18. This is of the rush kind that grows upon land, and are many sorts, but the sort that I shall here recommend is the bushy top jointed everywhere, resembling a horsetail, from whence it took its name. It is very powerful to staunch blood whenever, either inward or outward. A decoction of the herb being drank, it stops all manner of fluxes, and heals inward ulcers. It is good to heal a green wound, it cures ruptures in children, and it does ease the inflammation in the fundament.

ST. JOHN'S WORT.

19. It is well known that John's wort is a singular wound herb as any other whatever, either inward wounds, hurts or bruises, to be boiled in wine and drank, or prepared into oil or ointment,

bathe or taken inwardly. It has power to open obstructions, to dissolve swellings, to close up wounds, and to strengthen the parts that are feeble. The decoction of the herb and flowers, but of the seeds especially, in wine, helps all manner of spitting and vomiting blood: be it by any vein broke inwardly, by bruises, falls, or whatever provokes the terms. Two drachms of seed made into powder and drank in broth, does expel choler, or congealed blood in the stomach; it is good for all kinds of agues. A decoction of the seed is good for the sciatica, falling sickness, and the palsy.

LIVER-WORT.

20. Common liver-wort grows close, and spreads upon the ground in moist, shadowy places; with many sad green leaves, as it were sticking flat, one upon another, very uneven, cut in on the edges and crumpled.

It is a singular good herb for all diseases of the liver, both to cool and cleanse it. It is a singular remedy to stay the spreading of the tetters, ring-worms, sores, and scabs. It is good against surfeits of the liver.

MALLOWS.

21. This herb grows in every country, and almost in every door yard. There are two sorts of mallows, but their virtues are the same. A decoction of the herb and root, made in wine is opening to the body, and good in agues. A decoction of the seed made in milk, or wine, does marvelously help the phthisic, pleurisy, and other diseases of the chest. The juice drank in wine, or the decoction of them therein, does help women to speedy and safe delivery. Pliny said, that whoever drinks a spoonful of the juice in a morning, will be free from any disease that day. The leaves bruised and laid upon the eyes, takes the inflammation from them. The decoction of the leaves and roots, helps all sorts of poison; it is good for scabby heads, scalding, St. Anthony's fire, sore mouth, and throat. The green leaves bruised, with nitre, draw out thorns and prickles in the flesh. The high mallows is more effectual in all the before mentioned diseases.—The decoction of the leaves, is used in clisters, to ease all pains of the body, and open the passages. The decoction in white wine, is good for the king's evil, or swelling in women's breasts. A decoction of the root or juice, is good to give persons fainting, through loss of blood, and apply the same, mixed with honey and rosin, to the wound. Mallows bruised and boiled in milk, and the decoction for constant drink, boiled in water, cures the dysentary.

MOTHER-WORT.

22. This herb is so well known, that I shall not describe it. There is no better herb to drive melancholy vapors from the heart; to strengthen it, and make a merry, cheerful, blithe soul, than this herb is. Besides, it makes women joyful mothers, and regulates them after delivery, as they should be. The powder thereof, to the quantity of a spoonful, being drank in wine, is a wonderful help to women in sore travel. It is good for worms in children, it helps cramps, and convulsions.

SPEARMINT.

23. Spearmint has a healing, binding, and drying quality; and therefore, the juice taken in vinegar, checks bleeding. It is good to repress the milk in women's breasts. The bruised herb applied with salt, cures the bite of a mad dog. The often use use of the decoction, stays women's terms. It is good to wash the head of young children, that have breaking out sores, or scabs thereon. The powdered herb being taken after meat, helps bad digestion. Mint and worm wood, being boiled in but little water, and the herbs wet with spirits and bound on the bowels of the child, has a wonderful effect in bringing away worms.

MULLEN.

24. Mullen is well known. A small quantity of the root given in wine, is good against lax and fluxes. The decoction of th herb is good for those that are burst, for cramps, and convulsions, and for those that are troubled with an old cough. The decoction of the root in wine or water, is good against the ague; it opens obstructions of the bladder and reins, when one cannot make water.

Three ounces of the distilled water, drank morning and evening, for some days together, is a most excellent remedy for the gout. A decoction of the root and leaves, has great effect in dissolving the tumors, swelling, and inflammations of the throat. The seeds and leaves boiled in wine, and applied, draw forth speedily, thorns and splinters from the flesh, eases the pains and heals them. The same laid on any member newly sprained, or out of joint, or newly set, takes away all swelling and pain thereof.

MUSTARD.

25. This herb is very good in all diseases of the chest and lungs, hoarseness of voice, and by the use of decoction thereof, for a little space, those have been recovered, who had utterly lost their voice, and almost their spirits. It is good for coughs, shortness of breath, jaundice, the pleurisy, pains in the back and loins, for cholic, being also used in clisters. The seed is good against poison,

for the sciatica, gout and joint aches, sores, cankers in the mouth, throat, or behind the ears, for hard and swelled breasts.

HOARHOUND.

26. A decoction of the herb with the seed, or the juice of the green herb, taken with honey, is a sure remedy for those that are pursey, or short winded, or that have a cough, and are going into a consumption. The green herb boiled with milk, and a spoonful taken every morning, will restore a person far gone in the consumption. It is an excellent thing for women in travel, and for those that have taken poison. The leaves used with honey, are good for foul ulcers, and will stop running or creeping sores. The juice with wine and honey, helps to clear the eye-sight. The decoction is good for those that have bad livers; it kills worms, and is good for the asthma.

CATNIP, CATMINT, OR NEP.

27. The blows of catnip dried and powdered, and taken with honey for thirty days, is a certain cure for the phthisic. It is a good remedy; that is, the decoction of the herb for women to regulate their terms; it is good for pains in the head, catarrh, or dizziness thereof, and is used for colds, coughs, and shortness of breath. The juice made into an ointment and applied, is good for the piles.

NETTLES.

28. Nettle tops, eaten in the spring, consume the phlegmatic superfluities in the body of man, that the cold and moistness of winter has left behind. An electuary made of boiled roots, leaves or juice, is a safe and sure remedy to open the pipes and passages of the lungs; it is good to prevent the pleurisy: the same helps the swellings of the almonds of the ears and throat. The decoction in wine is good for women, and to open obstructions of the body. The decoction of the herb, or juice, or of the roots, is excellent to wash old rotten and stinking sores, fistulas, or gangrenes; it is of great use to bathe benumbed parts of the body, and gouty limbs.

WHITE-OAK.

29. The leaves and bark of the oak, are both binding and drying. The decoction of that bark and the powder of the cup that holds the acorn, will stay vomiting, and spitting of blood, bleeding at the mouth, and other fluxes of blood: the oak buds before they break out into leaves in decoction will do the same. The same is good in pestilential fevers, for it resists the force of the infection,

BOTANIC GARDEN.

it cools the heat of the liver. A decoction of the leaves is one of the best remedies for women's weaknesses that I know of.

OATS.

30. Oats fried with salt, and applied to the side takes away the pains. the meal of oats boiled in vinegar and applied, takes away freckles, and spots in the face, or other parts of the body.

ONIONS.

31. Onions being roasted in the embers, and eaten with honey and oil, do help an inveterate cough. The juice is good for a scald or burn; and used with vinegar, takes away all blemishes, spots, and marks of the skin; and dropped into the ears, eases the pains and noise in them. Leeks are wild and very common, and as good an herb as grows, to eat in the spring to physic the blood, and is an excellent guard against epidemical fevers, and other disorders. The root and herb, being boiled and applied, is an excellent remedy for the piles.

PARSLEY.

32. Parsley, a garden herb well known, is of an opening nature, and therefore good to open obstructions of the liver and spleen. It provokes urine mightily, especially if the roots be boiled and eaten like parsnips; is of course good for the gravel in the bladder; it is good to give children troubled with wind, and it takes away inflammation of the eyes. The herb being fried in fresh butter and applied to women's breasts, takes the pain, and swellings thereof. Take of the seeds of parsley, fennel, amsey and caraway, of each one ounce; of the roots of parsley, burnet, sassafras and caraway, of each an ounce and half; let the seeds be bruised and the roots washed and cut small; let them lie all night and steep in a bottle of white wine, and in the morning let them be boiled in a close earthen vessel, until a third part be evaporated which being strained and clear, take four ounces morning and evening, first and last, abstaining from drink after it the three hours. This will open obstructions of the liver and spleen and expel the dropsy and jaundice by urine.

SCABIOUS.

33. Scabious grows up with many hairy, soft, white, green leaves, some of which are but very little, if at all, jagged on the edges, others are very much rent and torn on the sides, and have threads in them, which, upon the breaking, may be plainly seen, from among which, rise up many hairy green stalks, three or four feet high, with such hairy green leaves on them; but more deeply and finely divided, and branched forth a little. At the tops thereof, which are naked and bare of leaves for a good space, stand round heads of flowers, of a pale bluish color, set together in a head.—The root is large and runs down into the ground, and of a reddish cast. It grows in meadows and in old fields and amongst corn. There are three or four sorts of scabious, but they are similar and their virtues are the same.

Scabious is very effectual for all sorts of coughs, shortness of breath, and all other diseases of the lungs and breast, ripening and digesting cold phlegm, and other tough phlegm, and humors, avoiding them by coughing and spitting. Drink the clarified juice in the morning, fasting, with a drachm of mithridate and molasses, frees the heart from infection, pestilence and epidemical complaints then let the party go to bed and sweat. The green herb pounded and applied to any bile or swelling, eases the pain and will draw it to a head. It helps all sores proceeding from the French disease. The juice of scabious, made up with the powder of borax and camphire, cleanses the face of freckles or pimples, and the head washed with the same cleanses away dandruff, scurf, sores, itch and the like. The bruised herb applied to the flesh, draws forth splinters, thorns, arrowheads, or the like, lying in the flesh.

SHEPHERD'S PURSE; OR SHEPHERD'S POUCH, TOY-WORT; OR CACE WEED.

34. This little herb has sundry names, and is an excellent pot herb. The root is small and white, and perishes every year. The leaves are small and long, of a pale green color, and deeply cut in on both sides, amongst which spring up a stalk which is small and round, with small leaves upon it even to the top, and the flowers are white, and very small.

It is of a dry, cold binding nature. It helps all fluxes, spitting of blood, and those that make bloody water, and being bound to the wrists and soles of the feet, it helps the yellow jaundice.—The herb made into a poultice, and applied, helps inflammations and St. Anthony's fire, and the juice dropped into the ear, eases the pain thereof.—A good ointment may be made of this herb for all wounds and especially those in the head.

COMMON SORREL.

35. Sorrel is a cooling herb, and therefore it helps inflammations and heat of blood in agues, sickness and fainting, and to refresh over spent spirits, that have had fits of fever and ague, and to quench thirst and cause an appetite in decayed stomachs. It resists the putrefaction of the blood, kills worms, and is a cordial to the heart. But the seed is most effectual, being more drying and binding. The roots, seeds and herbs, are good for the poison of a serpent.

A decoction of the flowers made in wine, helps the black jaundice and inward ulcers. A syrup made of the juice of sorrel and fumatory, is an excellent remedy to kill those sharp humors caused by the itch. The juice with vinegar and applied outwardly, is good for scald head or tetters, ring worms, &c. It helps the kernal in the throat and the juice is good for sores in the mouth. The herb pounded and roasted, being applied to a humour, hlotch or bite, will quickly fetch them to a head and break them.

WOOD SORREL.

36. Wood sorrel is of the same nature, and is good for all the aforementioned disorders, and is thought to be more effectual in hindering the putrefaction of the blood, and tempering inflammations. It is good to stay vomiting, and is excellent in pestilential and contagious fevers, cools inflammations in the throat, and helps them much.

STRAWBERRIES.

37. Strawberries when green are cold and dry, but when ripe are cold and moist. The berries are excellent to cool the liver blood and spleen, or any choleric stomach, fainting spirits, or quench thirst. They are not good to take in settled fevers. The leaves and roots boiled in wine and water, stays the bloody flux. The juice of the berries distilled, is a sovereign remedy for the panting and beating of the heart, and is good for the yellow jaundice. The juice, or the decoction of the herb or root, dropped into, or washed with the same, helps to cure foul ulcers, in any part of the body; is good to fasten loose teeth, and helps spungy and foul gums. The juice is good for inflamed and sore eyes; it is good for sores and humors on the body, redness of the face, or spots or other deformations of the skin, and will make it smooth and fair.

It is a very wholesome, cooling herb, and good with bread and milk; but to some people they are poison, and they cannot make any use of them whatever.

SMALL HOUSE-LEEK.

38. It grows with many trailing branches upon the ground, set with many thick, flat, roundish, whitish, green leaves, pointed at the ends. The flowers stand many of them together. It grows upon stone walls and mud walls; upon the tiles of houses and amongst rubbish; upon stumps or almost any place, with but little earth or moisture. It is of a cold nature and something binding, and therefore good to stay defluctions, especially such as fall upon the eyes. It expels poison, resists pestilential fevers, being exceeding good for tertian agues. You may drink the decoction of the herb for all the aforementioned diseases. It is so harmless an herb that you can hardly use it amiss. Being bruised and applied to the place, it helps the kings evil, and many other knots in the flesh, and also the piles.

TOBACCO.

39. Tobacco is found by experience to be good to expectorate tough phlegm from the stomach, chest and lungs. The juice is an excellent remedy for worms. You may sweeten, distill or make it into a syrup, and it answers the same purpose.—It eases the pain in the head, and the griping pains in the bowels. It helps to expel the stone in the kidney or bladder, and casts it off by urine. The seed thereof is very effectual to cure the toothache, and the ashes of the herb to cleanse the gums, and make the teeth white. The herb bruised and applied to the place aggrieved with the king's evil, is very effectual in nine or ten days. Manardas says it is a counter poison to any venomous serpent. The juice is good to kill lice in children's heads.

The juice applied to any green wound or cut, cures it very effectually, and will cleanse and heal old sores.

SPIGNARD; OR, PETIMORAL.

40. This is good in syrups for consumptive complaints. The roots boiled in wine or water, and drank, helps the stoppage of the urine, swellings and pains of the stomach, pains in the mouth, and all joint aches. If the powder of the root be taken with honey, it breaks tough phlegm, and dries up the rheum that falls upon the lungs. The roots are accounted very effectual against the sting or bite of any venomous creature. The roots pounded and applied to an old sore or wound, (the root must be boiled and the pith taken out,) will do wonders, when other things fail. The sore must be washed in the water in which the root was boiled, at every dressing.

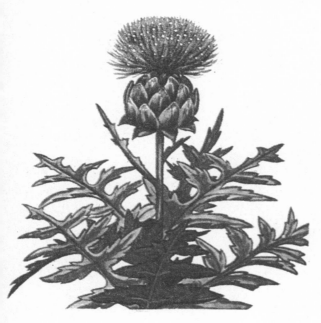

ARTICHOKE

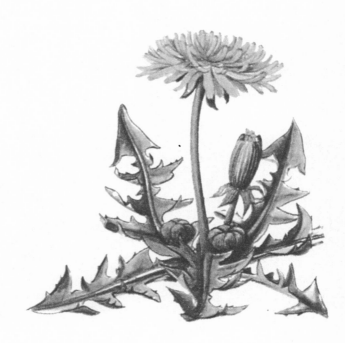

DANDELION

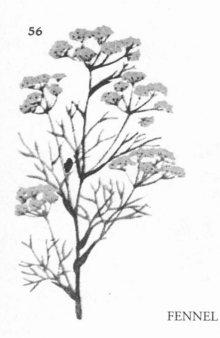

FENNEL

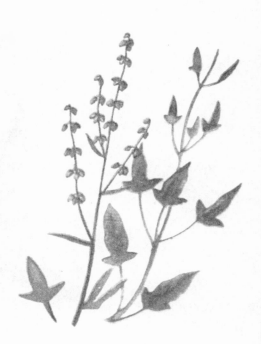

SORREL

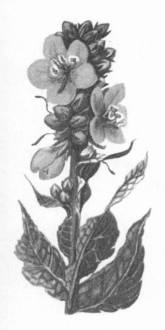

MULLEN

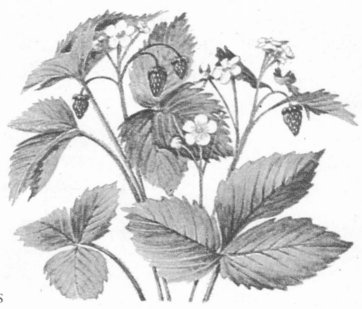

STRAWBERRIES

58

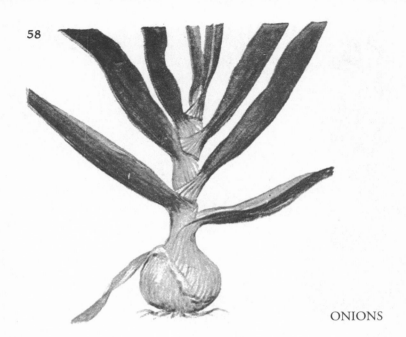

ONIONS

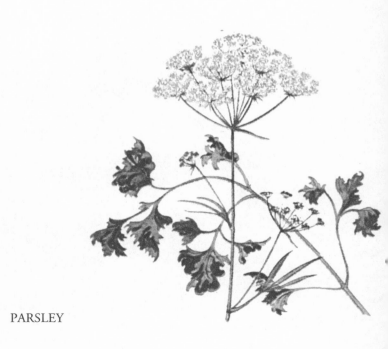

PARSLEY

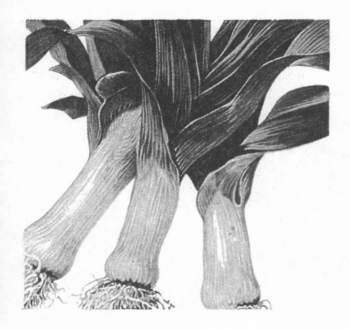

LEEK

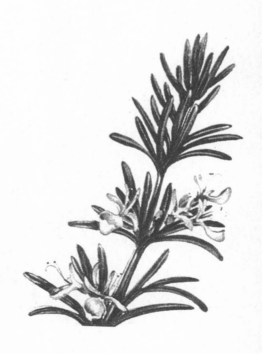

ROSEMARY

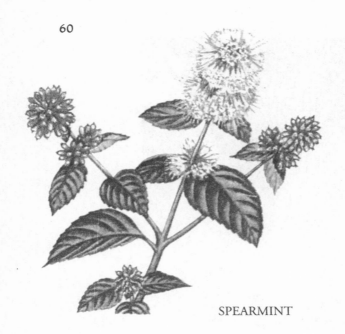

SPEARMINT

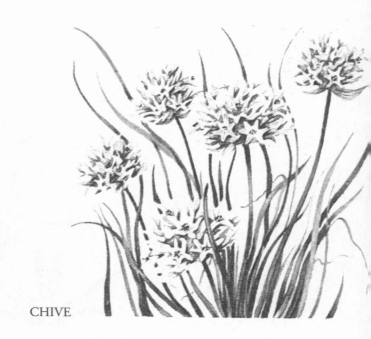

CHIVE